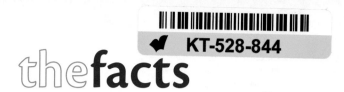

the**facts**

Infertility

MELANIE DAVIES
LISA WEBBER
CAROLINE OVERTON

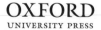

OXFORD
UNIVERSITY PRESS

OXFORD

UNIVERSITY PRESS

Great Clarendon Street, Oxford OX2 6DP

Oxford University Press is a department of the University of Oxford.
It furthers the University's objective of excellence in research, scholarship,
and education by publishing worldwide in

Oxford New York

Auckland Cape Town Dar es Salaam Hong Kong Karachi
Kuala Lumpur Madrid Melbourne Mexico City Nairobi
New Delhi Shanghai Taipei Toronto

With offices in

Argentina Austria Brazil Chile Czech Republic France Greece
Guatemala Hungary Italy Japan Poland Portugal Singapore
South Korea Switzerland Thailand Turkey Ukraine Vietnam

Oxford is a registered trade mark of Oxford University Press
in the UK and in certain other countries

Published in the United States
by Oxford University Press Inc., New York

© Oxford University Press 2009

The moral rights of the author have been asserted
Database right Oxford University Press (maker)

First published 2009

British Library Cataloguing in Publication Data
Data available

Library of Congress Cataloguing in Publication Data
Data available

Typeset in Plantin
by Cepha Imaging Pvt. Ltd., Bangalore, India
Printed in China
on acid-free paper by
Asia Pacific Offset

ISBN 978–0–19–921769–4 (Pbk.)

1 3 5 7 9 10 8 6 4 2

While every effort has been to ensure that the contents of this book are as complete, accurate
and up-to-date as possible at the date of writing, Oxford University Press is not able to give any
guarantee or assurance that such is the case. Readers are urged to take appropriately qualified
medical advice in all cases. The information in this book is intended to be useful to the general
reader, but should not be used as a means of self-diagnosis or for the prescription of medication.
The author and the publishers do not accept responsibility or legal liability for any errors in the
text or for the misuse or misapplication of material in this book.

Contents

Preface

This book is written for people who would like to know more about fertility, those who may have just discovered that there is a problem getting pregnant, and those who have been trying for some time. We aim to provide the facts about the body, fertility, and the different types of treatment available. This book covers all aspects of infertility—investigation, treatment, successful pregnancy, and coping with childlessness. Knowing the facts can reduce your worries about treatment and empower your choices. The book is in a plainspoken style; we have written as medical friends rather than as doctors. There are also details of reliable sources for more information and how to get help. The medical words are explained in the text and there is a glossary at the end of the book. We hope that this book helps you. If there is any additional information that would be useful for you in future editions, please let us know.

Melanie Davies
Lisa Webber
Caroline Overton

About the authors

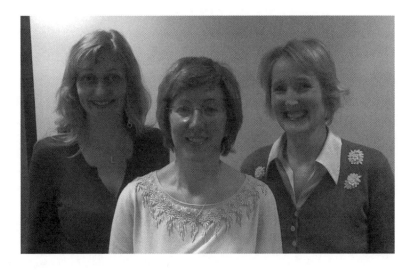

The three authors are all consultants in the UK specializing in fertility medicine and surgery. Melanie Davies is Consultant Obstetrician and Gynaecologist at University College Hospital, London. Her special interest is infertility and assisted conception, and she has worked in this field for 15 years. Lisa Webber is Consultant Gynaecologist at St Mary's Hospital, London, and her special interest is ovulation problems and polycystic ovary syndrome. Caroline Overton is Consultant Obstetrician and Gynaecologist at St Michael's Hospital, Bristol. Her special interest is endometriosis and laparoscopic surgery. We all met while working at University College London Hospital.

Contributing authors

Gerry Gajadharsingh is a qualified osteopath and diagnostic consultant of complementary medicine at The Health Equation in London (Chapter 9).

Jenny Clifford is a counsellor and psychotherapist who works in both primary care and the Assisted Conception Unit at University College London Hospital (Chapters 8 and 25).

Suks Minhas is Consultant Uro-andrologist and honorary senior lecturer at University College London Hospital (Chapters 10 and 23).

1

Overview of fertility and the biological clock

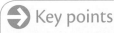 Key points

- About one in seven couples have difficulty in getting pregnant.
- Infertility is defined as the inability to get pregnant after more than 12 months of trying.
- A woman is born with her lifetime's supply of eggs within her ovaries.
- A woman's chances of getting pregnant decrease and her chances of miscarriage increase with advancing age.
- Men produce sperm continuously throughout their lifetime; from initiation to maturity takes about 64 days.

The female biological clock, age, and the chance of getting pregnant

You are not alone if you are having difficulty getting pregnant. It is estimated that one in seven couples have difficulty getting pregnant. Worldwide, 80 million couples have some difficulty in getting pregnant. Many couples prefer to keep this fact private, and so it is not until you start talking about your problems that you discover that some of your friends and family may be or have been in a similar situation.

It is a sad fact that some couples may never have a baby, yet there are many who go on to have a family successfully. For some couples, it is simply a question of time. For others, pregnancy may not happen. The uncertainty of whether pregnancy will or will not happen can add to the stress, with each month becoming a rollercoaster with every period. Unfortunately, there isn't a test that predicts if and when you will conceive.

It is normal to take up to 12 months to get pregnant, and sometimes up to 2 years without there being a problem. If you are young, your doctor may simply advise you to try a little longer.

You should be referred without delay if you or your partner are 35 or older, your period cycle is less than 26 days or more than 35 days, you don't have periods at all, you have had previous gynaecological problems such as **endometriosis**, **ectopic pregnancy**, or **pelvic infection**, or you have been trying for a baby for more than 3 years.

How long should it take to get pregnant?

If 100 couples (woman younger than 30) all decide to start trying for a family at the same time:

- 20 couples will be pregnant within the first month
- 70 couples will be pregnant within the first 6 months
- 85 couples will be pregnant within the first year
- 90 couples will be pregnant within the first 18 months
- 95 couples will be pregnant within the first 2 years

Doctors define **infertility** as the inability to get pregnant after 12 months of trying. **Primary infertility** is the term used for couples who have never conceived a pregnancy. **Secondary infertility** refers to couples who may have had a previous pregnancy either together or in a previous relationship.

To be able to understand why you may be having difficulty and what treatment involves, you will need to know some basic facts about the body.

The female biological clock

A woman is born with her lifetime's supply of egg sacs within her ovaries. These mature and ovulate, but no more are produced. This simple fact explains why women have a 'biological clock' and men don't. It also explains the increasing chance of having a baby with Down's syndrome as a woman approaches 40. This is an effect of ageing on the ovary and the eggs.

The chance of getting pregnant is reduced and the risk of miscarriage increases with age. That's not to say that older women will not get pregnant. Cherie Blair had Leo at the age of 45. The oldest woman recorded in the *Guinness Book of Records* to have a baby was 56, although there is some doubt about her age.

Age statistics

- Under the age of 30, the chance of miscarriage is one in five.
- Women aged 35–39 are half as fertile as they were at age 25.
- Women over the age of 40 are half as fertile as they were at age 35 and the chance of miscarriage is one in two.

However, these are only averages. Your own particular case is unique and will affect the chance of getting pregnant.

Men don't have a biological clock

Men produce sperm within the testicles throughout their lifetime. This is a continuous process. It takes about 64 days to produce a mature sperm. Men don't have a biological clock and can father children into old age. Several million sperm are present in a single ejaculate, yet it only takes one sperm and one egg to become pregnant (Figure 1.1).

Viral illnesses such as flu, smoking and alcohol, and exposure to certain chemicals and medicines reduce the number of sperm. Because of the production time, this effect is seen 3 months later. The testicles also like to be cool, and tight clothes or jobs involving long periods of sitting, such as long-distance lorry driving, may reduce sperm production. Some experts recommend that men wear loose-fitting underwear and trousers.

> ❌ **Myth:** Having too much sex reduces your chance of getting pregnant.

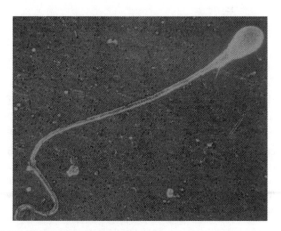

Figure 1.1 Magnified view of a mature sperm.

Working out the day of ovulation

Jan	Su	Mo	Tu	We	Th	Fr	Sa	
			(1)	(2)	(3)	(4)	(5)	January 1st is the first day of the period
	6	7	8	9	10	11	12	
	13	14	15	16	17	18	19	There are 28
	20	21	22	23	24	25	26	days until the next period
	27	28	(29)	(30)	(31)			[Ovulation day 14]

Feb	Su	Mo	Tu	We	Th	Fr	Sa	
						(1)	2	January 29th is the first day of the period
	3	4	5	6	7	8	9	
	10	11	12	13	14	15	16	There are 31 days
	17	18	19	20	21	22	23	until the next period
	24	25	26	27	28	(29)		[Ovulation day 17]

Mar	Su	Mo	Tu	We	Th	Fr	Sa	
							(1)	February 29th is the first day of the period.
	(2)	(3)	(4)	(5)	6	7	8	
	9	10	11	12	13	14	15	There are 28
	16	17	18	19	20	21	22	days until the next period.
	23	24	25	26	27	(28)	(29)	[Ovulation day 14]
	(30)	(31)						

Ovulation occurs between days 14 and 18 with 'fertile time' days 12–18.

Figure 1.2 Period diary showing cycle length and fertile time.

There are several tests on the market that enable a woman to detect when she is ovulating which can be bought over the chemist's counter. They involve testing the urine for a hormone called **luteinizing hormone** (see Chapter 7).

Once the egg is ovulated, it lives and can be fertilized for 24–48 hours. The man's sperm can stay alive and active for several days inside the woman's body. For this reason, it is better to have sperm 'ready and waiting' for the egg, rather than trying to time the exact day of ovulation. Avoid using lubricants. If you need a lubricant, choose one that is water (aqueous) based.

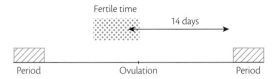

Figure 1.3 Your fertile time is the few days before ovulation. The number of days between the first day of your period and the day of ovulation will vary. The number of days between ovulation and a period starting (if you are not pregnant) is 14, give or take a day.

❌ **Myth:** You have to have sex exactly at the time of ovulation to get pregnant.

❗ **Fact:** Generally it is better to have sex as regularly and as often as possible when you are trying to get pregnant.

Your 'fertile time' is around ovulation. Sexual intercourse at other times in the month does not reduce your chances of pregnancy. Ovulation usually occurs 14 days before the expected period. This can be calculated in the following way.

You need to work out the number of days between your periods. Count the first day of your period as day 1. Work out the number of days between one period and the next. You may find that this number varies slightly. It is normal to have a period cycle of 26–35 days (Figure 1.2). Let us assume that you have a 30-day period cycle. The day of ovulation is usually 14 days before, give or take a day:

- for a 30 day cycle, the expected day of ovulation is day 16
- for a 34 day cycle, the expected day of ovulation is day 20
- and so on.

If you keep a temperature chart, your fertile time is the few days before your temperature rises (Figure 1.3).

In real life, the length of your period cycle may vary by a few days each month. This still means that you are ovulating. You can calculate the day of ovulation in your shortest and your longest cycle to know when your fertile time is.

It may seem as if you have been doing all of this, but still not getting pregnant. Not every egg is a good one and the sperm have to swim the equivalent of the Atlantic Ocean in treacle in order to fertilize the egg! Viewed this way, it is possible to see why pregnancy may take a little time to achieve.

2

Preparing for pregnancy

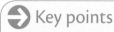 Key points

- Being overweight (defined as BMI > 30) reduces the chance of getting pregnant naturally by 50 per cent, even in women who ovulate regularly.

- Alcohol use can reduce fertility in both women and men. Drinking just 5 units of alcohol per week can mean that it will take you twice as long to get pregnant.

- Folic acid supplements taken around the time of conception and in early pregnancy can lower a woman's risk of having a baby with spina bifida (neural tube defect).

- Caffeine consumption may reduce fertility. World Health Organization guidelines suggest a maximum of two cups per day.

Looking after your general health is important, especially if you are planning a pregnancy.

◆ Try to eat a healthy balanced diet

A healthy balanced diet will nourish you and a developing baby. Eat five portions of fruit and vegetables per day and drink plenty of water.

◆ Try to lose weight if you are overweight

Do this by increasing the amount of exercise you do, as well as cutting down on the calories. Small regular meals are recommended. There are treatments available to assist you if you have already been trying to lose weight. Many primary care trusts do not fund NHS fertility treatment for women who are overweight, and this makes weight loss even more vital.

◆ **Your body mass index is important for fertility**

Your body mass index (BMI) is calculated as your weight in kilograms divided by your height in meters squared. The ideal body mass index is 19–24.9. A BMI of 25 or more is overweight and a BMI of 30 or more is obese (Figure 2.1). Most primary care trusts do not fund NHS fertility treatment for women with a BMI of more than 29:

$$BMI = \frac{\text{Weight (kilograms)}}{\text{height (metres)} \times \text{height (metres)}}$$

Your height-to-waist ratio is important for a healthy heart.

Being overweight (BMI over 30) halves the chance of getting pregnant naturally, even in women who are ovulating regularly. Losing weight helps in regulating periods (and ovulation) and the chance of a healthy pregnancy.

Overweight women respond less well to fertility drugs that are used for ovarian stimulation, although pregnancy rates are the same. Being overweight can affect the safety of fertility treatment, such as the ability to see the ovaries on ultrasound or a safe anaesthetic for laparoscopy or egg collection. Being overweight has a major impact during pregnancy and at delivery.

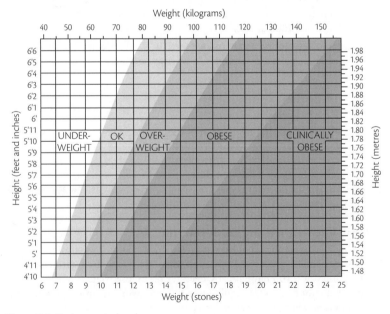

Figure 2.1 Body mass index chart.

There is an increased risk of miscarriage if you are overweight. This is also true in those who get pregnant by IVF or by donated eggs. Being overweight increases the risk of having a baby with a birth defect such as spina bifida, omphalocoele, or heart defects. This appears to be due to being overweight, but there also problems in seeing the baby clearly on scan if you are overweight.

Being overweight increases the chance of developing high blood pressure, venous thrombosis and diabetes during pregnancy. There is a higher chance of needing a Caesarean section, and being overweight makes the surgery more difficult. Wound infection is more common. The chance of the baby needing to be admitted to the special care baby unit is increased

◆ **Try to gain weight if you are underweight**

Being underweight can affect your monthly period cycle and even cause your periods to stop. Being underweight can also affect carrying the pregnancy with a smaller than average baby or premature delivery. Most fertility clinics insist that you are a normal weight before starting fertility treatment.

◆ **Speak to your doctor if you are taking any medicine(s) or have health problems**

For example, diabetes or high blood pressure. You need to be as healthy as possible for a pregnancy. Your doctor may want to change your medicine, because some medicines can be harmful to the developing pregnancy.

◆ **Speak to your doctor if there is a family history of a hereditary condition**

For example, cystic fibrosis or thalassaemia, for advice before you get pregnant.

◆ **Check with your doctor that you are up to date with your cervical smear**

Your doctor may also suggest a check for Chlamydia infection at the same time. Chlamydia infection can damage the Fallopian tubes. It sometimes has no symptoms.

◆ **Check with your doctor that you are immune to German measles (rubella)**

See your doctor for a test to check if you are immune to German measles (rubella). If caught during the first 3 months of pregnancy, this infection can harm your unborn baby. You can be vaccinated if you are not immune, but should not get pregnant for a month after the injection.

◆ **Stop smoking**

Tobacco contains toxic substances which may reduce fertility. Male fertility is affected by smoking as it decreases the sperm count, makes sperm more sluggish, increases the number of abnormal sperm, and reduces testosterone levels.

◆ **Cut down on your drinking**

Alcohol can affect your unborn baby, and can also reduce your fertility. This applies to men as well as women. Drinking just 5 units of alcohol per week can mean that it will take you twice as long to get pregnant. A unit is a small glass of wine, half a pint of normal strength beer, or a single measure of spirits.

◆ Take folic acid

Folic acid is a vitamin that is present in green vegetables and other foods. It has been found that women taking folic acid supplements around the time of conception and in early pregnancy have a lower risk of a baby with spina bifida (neural tube defect) which is an abnormality of the development of the brain and nervous system. These disorders are uncommon, but are important because babies can die or be severely handicapped as a result of them. The Department of Health has recommended that all women should take extra folic acid when they are trying to conceive and in the first 3 months of pregnancy. A daily vitamin supplement of 400 micrograms of folic acid is recommended. Folic acid can now be prescribed on the NHS or bought over a chemist's counter. Choose one specifically recommended for pregnancy. The cost of a 3 month supply is a few pounds. If you have previously had a child with neural tube defect or are taking medicine to control epilepsy, you need to increase the dose of folic acid.

◆ Try to keep a sensible work–life balance

Opinion is divided as to whether stress causes infertility. Your hormones are definitely affected by stress, anxiety, and tension. Some research suggests that stress makes the Fallopian tubes go into spasm and in men lowers the production of sperm.

◆ Strenuous exercise

Strenuous exercise appears to reduce the success of IVF treatment. Moderate exercise is good but needs to be a balance of relaxation, stretching, muscle strength, and cardiovascular exercise.

◆ Travel

Travelling a lot for your work will not affect your fertility, but being away from your partner may do so.

◆ The same health advice applies to the man

He should stop smoking, or at least cut down. He should reduce the amount of alcohol to a maximum of 2–3 units per night. If he is taking medicine, consult the doctor to make sure that these do not reduce sperm production.

◆ Recreational drugs

Marijuana, cocaine, heroin, ecstasy, and, in fact, almost all recreational drugs can reduce male and female fertility.

◆ Caffeine

Caffeine consumption may reduce fertility. The World Health Organization has issued caffeine guidelines (not just for subfertility), suggesting a maximum of 150 mg per day (equivalent to two cups of coffee).

3

Getting pregnant: a background to hormones and how the body works

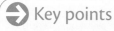 Key points

- Approximately one in five women attending a fertility clinic have a problem with ovulation, usually caused by a hormone imbalance.
- The hormones follicle-stimulating hormone (FSH) and luteinizing hormone (LH) control the development of eggs.

Hormones are chemicals produced by the body. They are produced by one part of the body and circulate in the bloodstream sending messages to other parts of the body. Several hormones are involved in the production of the egg and sperm.

About one in five women attending a fertility clinic have a problem with ovulation, usually caused by an imbalance in the hormones. Hormone drugs can be used to stimulate ovulation. An imbalance or shortage of hormones can also cause a problem with sperm production.

The female hormone cycle

Every month, several eggs start to develop in a woman's ovaries, but usually only one becomes fully mature and ovulates. The egg develops in a fluid-filled sac within the ovary called a follicle. Gonadotrophin-releasing hormone is produced by the hypothalamus in the brain and triggers the release of follicle-stimulating hormone (FSH) and luteinizing hormone (LH) from the pituitary gland, also in the brain (Figure 3.1).

These hormones produced by the pituitary gland control the development of the follicles. At the beginning of the period (menstrual) cycle, the pituitary gland releases follicle-stimulating hormone, which stimulates the ovary to produce follicles. One of these follicles grows faster than the others and is

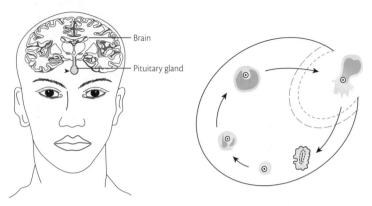

Figure 3.1 Development and release of an egg from the ovary (ovulation) is controlled by hormones produced by the brain. Reproduced from Vanderpump and Tunbridge, *Thyroid disease: the facts*, fourth edition (2008), with permission from Oxford University Press.

known as the 'dominant follicle'. It is from this follicle that an egg will be released (Figure 3.2)

The ovaries also produce hormones, one of which is called oestrogen. The developing follicle(s) produces oestrogen. Rising oestrogen levels stimulate the

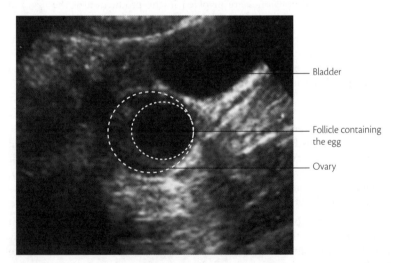

Figure 3.2 Ultrasound scan of a developing follicle inside an ovary. The follicle contains the egg.

pituitary gland to produce luteinizing hormone. When the level of luteinizing hormone peaks, it makes the ripest egg sac release the egg (ovulation).

Oestrogen stimulates the mucus produced by the cervix to become thin and slippery. Some (not all) women can see this change in the mucus and recognize when ovulation is happening. Some (not all) women get a pain in the ovary when the egg is released. This pain is called mittelschmerz.

The egg is picked up by the Fallopian tube, where it may be fertilized. When the egg sac (follicle) has released the egg, it changes to become a corpus luteum. Corpus luteum means 'yellow body'. This is because it looks yellow to the naked eye. The corpus luteum secretes the hormone progesterone.

In the first part of the cycle, (see figure 3.3) oestrogen produced by the ovaries stimulates the lining of the womb (endometrium) to thicken so that it is ready for the egg. Oestrogen makes the secretions produced by the neck of the womb become thin and slippery so sperm can easily swim through it (Figure 3.4).

Progesterone produced after ovulation makes the lining thick and juicy ready to nourish a fertilized egg and possibly a pregnancy will start. If a pregnancy does not start, the corpus luteum shrinks, progesterone levels fall, the lining of the womb is shed as a period, and the cycle begins again.

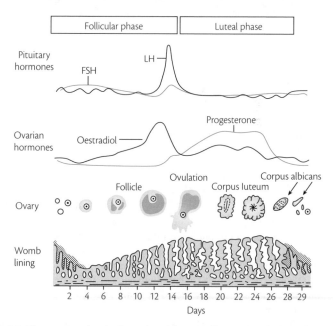

Figure 3.3 The menstrual cycle. Reproduced from Sanders *et al. Oxford Handbook for the Foundation Programme* (2005), with permission from Oxford University Press.

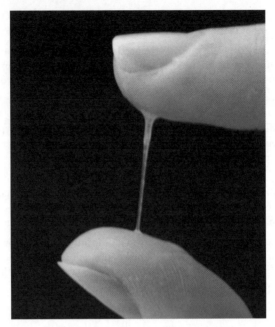

Figure 3.4 At the time of ovulation the cervical mucus changes to become thin and stretchy.

 Fact: Premenstrual symptoms indicate that ovulation has happened. The hormone progesterone produced after ovulation causes breast tenderness, moodiness, and water retention.

The womb, tubes, and ovaries

The womb (uterus) is a pear-shaped organ in the centre of the pelvis. It is approximately the size of a small pear, and is about 7 or 8 centimetres long. The womb is attached to the vagina and the entrance of the womb (cervix) can be seen in the upper vagina. The two Fallopian tubes are smaller in diameter than your little finger. They are attached to the upper part of the womb, one on each side. The ends of the tubes are trumpet-shaped and fringed, and open into the abdominal cavity near the ovaries. The ovaries are two plum-sized glands attached to the womb (Figure 3.5).

In the textbooks, the drawings show the tubes sticking out at right angles from the womb. In life, they are much softer and dangle behind the womb in a pocket

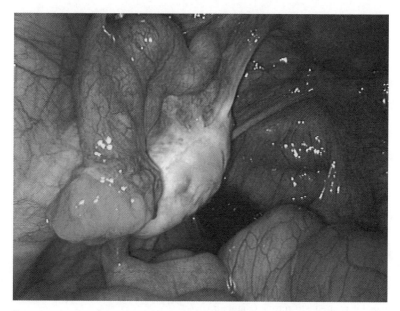

Figure 3.5 Laparoscopic picture of a normal Fallopian tube and ovary.

known as the pouch of Douglas or the cul de sac. This pocket is important, because it is from here that the egg is picked up.

  Myth: A retroverted uterus means that you can't get pregnant.

Fact: The uterus always tilts, usually forwards (anteverted) but sometimes backwards (retroverted). A healthy retroverted uterus does not prevent pregnancy.

The testicles

The testicles are two plum-sized glands found in the scrotum. The testicles are designed to be outside the body because they work better at lower temperatures. The same hormones that control stimulation of the ovary stimulate the release of testosterone and also sperm production. Gonadotrophin-releasing hormone is produced by the hypothalamus in the brain and triggers the release of follicle-stimulating hormone and luteinizing hormone from the pituitary gland. Follicle-stimulating hormone stimulates sperm production in

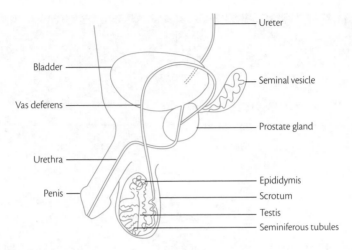

Figure 3.6 Male anatomy.

the testicles, while luteinizing hormone stimulates the testicles to produce the male hormone testosterone (Figure 3.6).

Sperm travel from the testicles to the epididymis, a long coiled tube. The sperm mature as they travel through the epididymis. From the epididymis, they pass down the vas deferens to the penis. When a couple have sex and the man 'comes' or ejaculates, the sperm are forced from his penis into the vagina in powerful spurts.

> ❌ **Myth:** You don't have to have sex on your back to get pregnant.
>
> ❌ **Myth:** A lot of women worry that the sperm trickle out after sex.
>
> ❗ **Fact:** This is the liquid that carries the sperm. Sperm move quickly through the cervix and can be seen inside the body a few minutes after sex!

4

How to choose your clinic

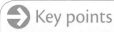 **Key points**

◆ The GP is the first port of call for couples seeking fertility investigations
  and treatment. Your GP should refer you to a fertility specialist.

◆ Try having your initial investigations in your local NHS fertility clinic.
  Not all areas will fund all forms of fertility treatment and you may have
  to fund your own treatment at some stage.

◆ An increasing number of UK-based couples now seek fertility treatment
  abroad because of lower treatment costs and ease of obtaining donor
  eggs/sperm.

For most couples wanting to embark on fertility investigations and treatment,
the first place to start is with your general practitioner (GP). Assuming that you
are eligible for NHS treatment, it is worth having the initial investigations in
your local NHS fertility clinic, especially since not all primary care trusts
(PCTs) will fund all forms of fertility treatment and you may have to consider
funding your own treatment at some stage. Your GP will be able to refer you to
the appropriate specialist and will be able to advise you on how long you can
expect to wait for that appointment. You should ensure that you have been
referred to a specialist who has a particular interest in fertility problems and
their treatment. Do make sure that both of you are registered with a GP and
take the details of your GP(s) (i.e. name, address, telephone number) to your
first appointment.

Even if you are planning to see a doctor privately it is still worth discussing your
plans with your GP as the fertility clinic will ask for your permission to contact
him or her should you require a treatment that is licensed by the Human
Fertilisation and Embryology Authority (HFEA) (see Chapter 5). A small

number of GPs are able to partially fund the cost of private fertility treatment by prescribing the drugs for you.

Most GPs will offer to arrange basic investigations, and whether these are done before a referral is made or while you are waiting to be seen by the specialist will depend on your age, how long you have been trying to have a baby, and any relevant medical history. See Chapter 7 for a detailed discussion of fertility investigations and their timings.

It may be that your local NHS fertility clinic is able to provide the type of treatment that you require. However, more complex treatments such as IVF and IVF-related treatments may require referral from your local clinic to another unit. If you are having NHS-funded treatment you are unlikely to have a choice in where you are referred as it will depend on where your PCT has arranged its contract. It may be that the type of treatment you require, or your circumstances (e.g. your age, or that one of you has been sterilized) means that you are not eligible for treatment funded by your PCT. This may mean that you decide to pay for your own treatment. Sometimes, the wait for NHS treatment may be unacceptably long for you and so you may choose to pay for private treatment. This may be particularly worth considering if you are a woman over 38 years old and are facing a delay of over a year.

How do I find out about clinics in my area?

Your GP may be able to provide you with the names of local clinics and doctors. It is always worth asking for your GP's recommendations as the chances are that he or she will have other patients who have had similar problems. It may be that you know someone who was seen in a particular clinic and you would (or would not!) like to be seen there as a result of that person's experience. However, it is important to remember that your situation may be different from your friend and therefore a different unit may be more appropriate for you (see below).

A list of clinics offering licensed fertility treatment in your area is available from the HFEA's website (see Useful addresses). There are over 80 such clinics in the UK; London and the North East are best provided for, and the North West and Wales have the lowest number of fertility clinics per patient population.

How do I choose a clinic for the initial investigations?

The most important consideration when you are looking for a clinic for the initial investigations is that you are being seen by a doctor who has a special interest in fertility problems. At this stage it does not really matter whether or not the clinic in which this doctor is based offers all forms of fertility treatments, especially since many couples conceive during the initial investigations!

The clinic you are going to should have easy access to the necessary specialist investigations within an acceptable length of time. Similarly, you should be able to have follow-up appointments without undue delay. Remember that most investigations need to be carried out over at least one menstrual cycle and it is best to complete these before your next consultation.

Fertility investigations usually involve attending for tests at certain times in the menstrual cycle, and so choosing a clinic that is geographically convenient to attend can be important and may make the process less stressful.

How do I choose a clinic for fertility treatment?

The obvious main consideration here is that the clinic should be able to provide the type of treatment you require within a timescale that is appropriate and acceptable for your circumstances. Unless you require highly specialized treatment such as preimplantation genetic diagnosis (PGD) (see Chapter 16), you are likely to have a choice of more than one clinic. Again, geographical proximity of the clinic to your home or place of work should be a consideration as you are likely to be required to attend for tests, such as ultrasound scans and or blood tests, perhaps as frequently as every 2 days once your treatment has started.

If you are having a treatment that is regulated by the HFEA (see Chapter 5), the pregnancy and live birth rates for individual clinics are published by the HFEA (see Useful addresses). However, these figures (often referred to as 'league tables') do have to be interpreted with care. For example, a clinic with a seemingly low pregnancy rate may simply be less selective about the couples they treat than another clinic with an apparently higher rate, or the average ages of the women treated may be different (higher pregnancy rates being seen when women are younger).

Most private fertility units will be able to send you a brochure about the services they offer and many run 'open days' when you can visit and meet some of the professionals who will be involved in your care. This is a good opportunity to ensure that you feel comfortable with the way in which the clinic works and perhaps to ask specific questions about the sort of treatment you may need. Some couples may feel more comfortable in a smaller unit where they will see the same professionals throughout their treatment, whereas this may be less important for other couples. If you have to travel a considerable distance to the clinic, it may be important that your appointments can be at a time that allows for this.

How do I choose a clinic that is overseas?

An increasing number of UK-based couples are seeking fertility treatment overseas. This may be because treatment costs are lower in certain countries, but the main driving force is the need to use donor eggs or sperm. In some countries the laws governing the recruitment and payment of egg and sperm donors are different and therefore they are easier to obtain. In the UK, the HFEA regulates treatment (discussed in detail in Chapter 5). However, it has no role in overseas treatment, even when this has been arranged via a UK-based clinic. If you are thinking about treatment abroad, you should consider carefully factors such as the quality control of the treatments offered, confidentiality, possible legal implications of treatment, particularly when donor eggs or sperm are used, and any ethical issues surrounding the recruitment of donors. In the UK both donors and recipients are required to receive independent counselling to explore possible consequences of donation or treatment; this is not so in all countries.

More and more UK clinics are forging links with overseas clinics to make treatment more accessible. Overseas treatment can be very successful, particularly in the context of requiring an egg or sperm donor of ethnic minority in the UK. It is vital that before committing to treatment, you consider all aspects and implications of treatment and it is advisable to seek the experience of other couples who have been treated in the country you are considering. A link to the websites of patient organizations in various countries is available from Infertility Network UK's website (see Useful addresses).

5

The law and fertility treatment (regulation)

⮕ Key points

- In the UK all fertility treatment is regulated by the Human Fertilisation and Embryology Authority (HFEA).
- HFEA protects those seeking licensed treatments by ensuring that clinics work to the standards set by the regulator. Clinics undergo regular inspections by HFEA officers in order to gain and renew their licenses.
- Regulation of fertility treatment internationally varies from country to country and, in some cases, between regions within a country.
- When obtaining fertility treatment abroad, it is important to consider carefully regional variations in fertility regulations.

Fertility treatment in the UK is regulated by the Human Fertilisation and Embryology Authority (HFEA) which is a statutory body created by the Human Fertilisation and Embryology Act 1990. No other branch of medicine in any country in the world is controlled to such an extent by a governing body or, indeed, by a specific Act of Parliament. If you have a consultation in an HFEA licensed clinic (see below) some of the forms you will be asked to complete will be at the requirement of the HFEA. Certain treatments (currently those related to IVF) carry a fee levied by the HFEA which you will have to pay in addition to your treatment costs if you are having private care.

The Act came about after the first successful IVF treatment which was performed in 1977 and resulted in the birth of Louise Brown on 25 July 1978. At the time the treatment was highly controversial, although by the time Louise was born 5000 couples had expressed an interest in receiving treatment. The main debate surrounded the rights of the embryo and the ethics of manipulating a potential human being. After much public discussion, the Committee of

Inquiry into Human Fertilisation and Embryology, whose chair was Baroness Warnock, published its report in 1984 and the Act followed 6 years later.

The main purpose of the HFEA when it was first created was to guard against experimentation on embryos. For example, the Act limits the time that an embryo can be kept alive outside the body to 14 days, which is when the rudimentary nervous system (the primitive streak) first develops. Three decades on from the first successful IVF treatment and almost a decade into a new century, the HFEA now regulates all forms of fertility treatment which involve the manipulation of gametes (eggs or sperm, including immature gametes within testicular or ovarian tissue). Such treatments can only be performed by assisted conception centres which have been granted a licence by the HFEA. These are called 'licensed centres'.

Licensed treatment

- IVF—all forms
- Gamete intra-Fallopian transfer (GIFT)
- Intrauterine insemination (IUI)
- Donor insemination (DI)
- Use of donor eggs
- Storage of eggs/sperm
- Storage of embryos
- Research involving fresh eggs/sperm
- Research involving embryos

Part of the statutory duty of the HFEA is to collect information about licensed treatment from all licensed centres; these data are published as live birth rates by the HFEA and are often referred to as 'league tables'. The latest figures are obtainable from the HFEA and are published annually on their website (see Useful addresses).

Implications of attending a licensed centre

All licensed centres have to abide by the high standards laid out in the Code of Practice produced and regularly updated by the HFEA. Thus the HFEA protects embryos, gametes, and couples seeking and undergoing licensed treatments.

Confidentiality

Individuals or couples undergoing any form of fertility treatment are assured that confidentiality will be maintained in the same way as for any form of medical consultation or treatment. However, those undergoing licensed treatment are assured of additional confidentiality: details of licensed treatment, including the proposal to perform licensed treatment, can only be disclosed to others not covered by a licence with the written permission of those being treated. This means that you can expect to be asked to sign a form giving your permission to keep your GP informed of your treatment; this is usually called 'Consent to Disclosure' and your clinic may well use the form produced by the HFEA for the purpose.

If you are a couple seeking treatment, both of you will be asked to give your consent. Usually, information is disclosed to the female partner's GP. Generally, it is in your own best interest to allow the clinic to keep your GP informed; however, you may prefer that certain aspects of your treatment are not mentioned and you will be given an opportunity to specify this on the consent form. You will be asked for the reason why you do not wish to give this information.

You will also be asked if you consent to passing information to other medical staff who are not covered by an HFEA license; this is for continuity of your care. The two final questions on consent you will be asked are whether you would allow your details to be included in an audit of treatment or an accounts audit (this last group really only applies if your treatment is within a private clinic).

Many clinics ask that you complete these forms on your first visit and some will actually send them to you at home before your first appointment, even before it is known whether or not you require treatment that is covered by a licence.

Welfare of the child

A licensed centre has a duty to take into account the impact of treatment on the mental and physical wellbeing of any existing or potential children. This has to be done fairly and without prejudice. Most clinics will ask that you complete a brief self-assessment form for this purpose; again, it is often one produced by the HFEA. All individuals or couples attending a licensed clinic have to undergo some form of 'welfare of the child' assessment, and the HFEA encourage licensed clinics to make their assessment at the first visit. Paradoxically, if you are referred to a clinic that does not perform licensed treatment, you will not have to undergo this assessment.

It is very rare that a clinic would need to withhold treatment because of concerns under this heading. Certainly, any decision to do so must be taken very seriously and after consultation within the unit involved. If you are refused treatment, you can expect to have the reasons explained and the steps required, if any, that would change the decision of the clinic. You should also be given an opportunity to appeal. Your consent or otherwise for disclosure to your GP may be taken into consideration when this sort of decision has to be made.

Examples of factors that *may* lead to treatment being refused

- Previous convictions relating to harming children
- Child protection measures taken regarding existing children
- Serious violence or discord within the family
- Circumstances likely to lead to an inability to care for the potential child throughout childhood (e.g. physical or mental conditions or substance abuse)

This role of the HFEA is understandably controversial as society does not have the right to 'regulate' who is able to become a parent when the pregnancy is spontaneous. Some feel that this amounts to discrimination against couples with fertility problems. It may be that this requirement will be dropped in the future.

What does the HFEA do?

The HFEA protects those seeking licensed treatments by ensuring that clinics work to the standards set by the regulator. These standards cover all aspects of treatment, from patient information documents to air quality within the laboratory and everything in between. Clinics undergo regular inspections by HFEA officers in order to gain and renew their licence.

The HFEA maintains and publishes a list of all licensed clinics within the UK along with each clinic's live birth rates for the various treatments offered. It is also possible to view the latest inspection report for each clinic. A central register of donor information is also maintained; since April 2005 this has included identifying information. The offspring of donor treatment can obtain these details when they reach the age of 18 years.

Complaints against clinics can be made to the HFEA, although every clinic must have a complaints process which should be publicized within the unit.

Finally, the HFEA publishes a free booklet for those seeking treatment. It is updated annually and is a very useful overview of different aspects of infertility and its treatment. In addition, there is much useful information on the HFEA website, together with links to other relevant sites.

Regulation internationally

There is no pan-European regulation of fertility treatment, but the European Union Tissues and Cells Directive is relevant to certain aspects of treatment. As of July 2007, all member states must comply with this Directive which stipulates the standards that must be adhered to when handling, processing, or storing human tissues and cells that are for human use.

Regulation of fertility treatment internationally varies from country to country and sometimes between regions within a country. Some couples may specifically seek treatment abroad to take advantage of these variations. A common example is egg or sperm donation; many couples prefer to have an anonymous donor and therefore choose to have their treatment in a country where donor anonymity is guaranteed (e.g. Denmark and Spain). In some countries, including the UK and Sweden, only eggs and sperm from identified donors can be used for treatment (even if the eggs/sperm are 'imported'), and the donors' details are kept on a secure national register (see above). Other couples may feel that they have to travel for their treatment if it is not available locally. Currently, the most common reason for overseas treatment for UK-based couples is donor treatment because of a lack of UK donors (both for eggs and for sperm).

It is very important to consider issues such as these if you are considering treatment abroad. There may also be local legal issues related to certain forms of treatment (particularly surrogacy), and it may be appropriate to seek independent legal advice before embarking on treatment. At the moment there is no central information point regarding treatment in different countries, but Infertility Network UK (see Useful addresses) have a link on their website to patient organizations in various countries which can be a useful resource.

Issues to consider if having treatment abroad

- Will my treatment be confidential?
- Are the clinic's live birth rates available and, if so, are they up to date and verified?
- Are there any local legal implications of my treatment (e.g. if donor eggs or sperm are used, or if it involves surrogacy)?
- If using donor eggs or sperm, has the donor been screened for infectious diseases (eg hepatitis B, hepatitis C, HIV, Chlamydia) and inherited diseases?
- Is my egg/sperm donor anonymous or will my potential child be able to find out any information regarding their genetic parentage?
- If donor information is kept, how long is it kept for, how is confidentiality maintained, and what happens to that information if the clinic closes?
- Can the offspring of donor treatment be reassured that they are not unwittingly forming an intimate relationship with a relative?
- What information will I be given regarding my donor (e.g. ethnic background, physical characteristics, education, employment)?

- How are donors recruited and under what circumstances?
- How many offspring can any one donor produce, or is there no regulation?
- How many embryos can be transferred at any one time? Can I be involved in the decision?

The future

At the time of writing, the Human Fertilisation and Embryology Act 1990 is under government review, which will undoubtedly bring some changes to the regulation of fertility treatment. It is not expected that the new Act will lessen the principles of regulation laid down in the original Act.

6

The initial consultation: what is covered in your first clinic visit?

➜ Key points

- The main aim of the initial consultation is to perform a medical assessment of you and your partner.

- Both you and your partner will be asked to answer a series of questions relating to your general health, to identify any health problems that might affect a pregnancy.

- Most women will be examined during their first clinic visit including a vaginal examination.

- The doctor will explain which tests are recommended and why, and may offer some suggestions for improving the chances of conception.

The aim of your first visit to the fertility clinic is a medical assessment of you and your partner in order to plan your initial investigation and treatment. Most clinics prefer both partners to attend at least one visit together, and if this is difficult, it is probably most useful if it can be this first one. Don't be put off if your appointments are only addressed to one of you; most clinics traditionally keep fertility records under the name of the woman. Rest assured that your partner will be most welcome at all times!

It is important that the clinic can contact you, and the clinic receptionist will check your personal details (address, telephone numbers, and GP details) at each visit. It is in your best interests to keep the clinic informed of any changes to these details.

Medical questions

The doctor will start by asking you a series of questions about yourself, your partner, and your lifestyle. This is called a medical history. The questions aim to identify any health problems that might affect a pregnancy and to improve your health. These may include, for example, advice to stop smoking, a check that you are immune to rubella (also known as German measles), and a recommendation to take preconception folic acid (see Chapter 2).

Fertility questions

The first group of questions usually includes a question about how long you have been trying to get pregnant. The doctor will enquire about any previous pregnancies, including those within a previous relationship. He/she will make a note of what the outcomes were and if there were any complications: for example, if you had an infection, needed a repeat operation (often referred to as a D&C or ERPC to remove a miscarried pregnancy), or any problems during pregnancy, such as premature labour or diabetes.

Whilst it is in your best interest to provide frank answers to such questions, you may have had a previous pregnancy that you would prefer your partner not to know about. There is usually an opportunity to discuss such matters in confidence with your doctor, if not during your first visit, then at a later one. (Your GP will probably know about a previous pregnancy and mention it in your referral letter to the clinic. If you would prefer that it is not discussed in front of your partner, you can ask your GP to state that in the letter.)

If you have had fertility investigations or treatment before, even with a different partner, it is very helpful to bring details with you. If possible, these should include the types of any investigations, their results, and what, if any, treatments you underwent. While you are waiting for your first appointment to arrive, you could use this time to contact your previous clinic directly to request that these details are sent to you.

Gynaecological questions

It would be helpful if you have the following information with you.

- How many days between the first day of one period and the first day of the next period (the menstrual cycle) (see Chapter 1).

- How many days you bleed for, whether the flow is particularly heavy or light, and if you experience period pain.

- The date of your last menstrual period (also known as LMP).

- The year and result of your last cervical smear.

- Details of any ongoing or previous gynaecological problems (including past pelvic infections, also known as pelvic inflammatory disease or PID) and operations.

You can expect to be asked for basic details of your sex life—don't be embarrassed, everyone attending a fertility clinic has one! Your doctor will enquire about how often you make love (have sexual intercourse) and any particular problems you may have such as pain, difficulty with penetration, or bleeding afterwards. He/she will also want to know if your partner has problems achieving or maintaining an erection or reaching orgasm.

General questions

Part of the medical history includes questions about your general health. This includes details of current or previous medical problems (e.g. asthma, diabetes, a clot in your leg or lung) as well as previous operations. Your doctor will be interested in any operations you may have had, even if they were not gynaecological. You will also be asked about any tablets or medicines you take, any allergies you have (including food or skin allergies), and whether you smoke, drink alcohol (if so, how much), or use any other recreational drugs (e.g. cannabis, cocaine, ecstasy, heroin, etc).

Questions for the man

Your partner can expect to be asked similar questions to those outlined above, except that details of any testicular problems would replace the gynaecological details! Specifically, these would include trauma or surgery to the genitals, hernia repair, and any previous infections.

Examination

Most women will be examined at their first clinic visit, although if you are having your period this can be postponed to a later visit. Examination usually includes feeling the tummy (palpating the abdomen) and a vaginal examination. The latter involves gently inserting one or two fingers into the vagina in order to feel the size of the womb (uterus), and the presence of any swellings or tender areas. A plastic or metal speculum is generally also used in order to visualize the vagina and cervix (similar to when a smear is taken). Some doctors will also include a breast examination at this visit.

Many doctors will only examine the man if a particular problem has been identified, for example if the sperm count is found to be low or abnormal swellings are reported.

Variations you may encounter

Some clinics may ask you and your partner to complete a questionnaire before you see the doctor. This might be sent to you before your appointment, you may be asked to fill it in at the clinic when you are waiting to see the doctor, or you may see a nurse who will take these details from you first. A few clinics may request that your GP arranges some basic tests and that you bring the results of these with you to your first appointment.

What to expect after all the questions

The answers that you give to your doctor's questions, together with the findings when you are examined, will help your doctor to tailor the investigations to your own particular circumstances. Usually the first consultation ends with a summary of any potential causes for your delayed conception that have been identified. The doctor will then explain which tests are recommended and why (these are discussed in the next chapter). He/she may also make some recommendations that may help you to conceive, for example on the optimum frequency and timing of sexual intercourse, or any lifestyle changes that may be beneficial.

Finally, this is, of course, an opportunity for you and your partner to ask questions and to address any specific concerns you may have. Most doctors welcome this opportunity, as involvement in your own care can relieve stress and may improve outcomes.

Summary of questions you can expect

Questions for both partners

- How long you have been trying to have a baby.
- How long you have been together.
- Details of previous pregnancies (including those from previous relationships).
- Previous and current medical problems.
- Previous operations.
- Names of any medicines you may be taking.
- Any allergies, particularly to medicines.
- If you smoke, how many cigarettes per day?
- If you drink alcohol, how many units in a week?
- If you use any recreational drugs.
- How often you have sex.
- If you have any problems with intercourse.
- Medical information about members of your family (parents, siblings, any existing children).

Questions for the woman

- When your last period *started* (last menstrual period (LMP))
- How often your period comes.
- Any problems you may have with your periods.
- Any bleeding from the vagina between your periods or after intercourse?
- Is sex painful or difficult for you?
- When was your last smear?

Questions for the man

- Any injuries to the testes in the past?
- Any operations particularly hernia repair or surgery to the genitals.
- Any episodes of testicular pain or swelling, past or present?
- Any difficulties with intercourse—achieving or maintaining an erection or with ejaculation?

7

Why aren't I getting pregnant? Fertility tests

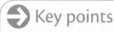 Key points

- Most couples are advised to have tests after a year of trying for a baby.
- Couples who have normal tests after a year of trying have a 50 per cent chance of conceiving during the next year.
- Ovulation tests for the hormone LH are available over the counter and can be done at home without seeing a doctor.
- Men will be asked to provide a semen sample for analysis. If the initial results are not good they will be asked to give another sample in a few weeks.
- Try to see an experienced doctor or nurse to go through the results of your tests fully.

When are tests needed?

Couples are usually advised to have tests after a year of trying for a baby. After a year, most healthy couples will have conceived (see Chapter 1 for an overview of fertility). The tests may well show an unexpected problem which explains the delay in getting pregnant. Once you know what the problem is, you can then move on to treatment and hopefully a successful pregnancy.

If the tests are all normal, you can be reassured that nothing is seriously wrong. You have probably been unlucky so far, and can still get pregnant naturally. Couples who have normal tests after a year of trying will have a 50 per cent (1 in 2) chance of conceiving during the next year.

Tests should be done earlier if either partner has a medical history that could cause infertility. For example, if the man has a history of operations on the testicles, the sperm count may be low; if the woman had an ectopic pregnancy in the past, her tubes may be damaged; if she has very irregular periods, she may not be releasing eggs. More details are given in Chapter 6.

If the woman is aged over 35, tests should be done in less than a year. Fertility decreases with age in women, and treatment should be started promptly.

Overview of fertility tests

The list of tests to be done may seem very long, and it can be dispiriting to make many visits to the clinic. However, if they are carried out efficiently, all the basic tests can be done within a few weeks and most of them within one menstrual cycle.

The tests are designed to answer the following three basic questions:

- Are there enough healthy sperm?
- Are healthy eggs being produced?
- Can the eggs and sperm meet?

Your list of tests may look complicated, but they fall into these groups. They are described in detail in the rest of this chapter.

Home testing

Some tests can be done at home without seeing a doctor. You can monitor your menstrual cycle by writing down the days on which your period starts and working out the length of the cycle (see Chapter 1). If the cycle length is 26–35 days then you are almost certainly ovulating. The egg is released 14 days before the period starts. You may notice that the vaginal secretion is wetter, clearer, and more slippery for a few days before ovulation. This is mucus made by the cervix, which can hold the sperm for at least 2 days. Being aware of this can help you to conceive, as making love just before ovulation gives you the highest chance of pregnancy.

Measuring your body temperature can also show whether you are ovulating. In the second half of the monthly cycle, a woman's 'basal' body temperature is a little higher (half a degree Celsius). Your temperature needs to be taken every day first thing in the morning, before you get out of bed, and before having a hot drink. If you chart your temperature every day, it should dip down slightly just at the time of ovulation and then rise (Figure 7.1). The problem with temperature charts is that they are often hard to interpret, for example you may have a rise in temperature because of a sore throat, and they only show ovulation in hindsight. Nowadays, most doctors do not recommend temperature charts.

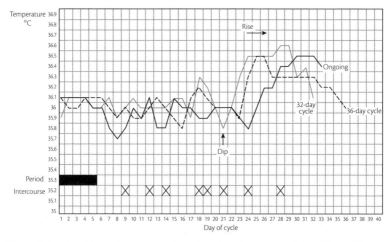

Figure 7.1 A basal body temperature chart showing a long cycle of 32–36 days with a slightly short luteal phase.

Ovulation tests for the hormone LH are available over the counter. These can pinpoint the day of ovulation more accurately than a temperature chart. Moreover, they give advance warning of ovulation so that you can make love at your most fertile time. Several kits which test urine for the presence of LH are available. Each kit contains several test strips which change colour or show a symbol such as a smiling face (Figure 7.2). A positive result predicts that the

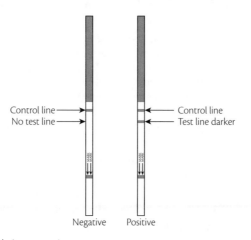

Figure 7.2 Ovulation test strips.

35

egg will be released 24–36 hours later. These tests are accurate for most women, but will not be helpful if you have a very long or irregular cycle. Also, they occasionally give false results if women have high LH levels all the time (this can happen with PCOS or early menopause).

A more sophisticated version of ovulation testing at home measures two hormones, LH and oestradiol, to indicate the fertile 'window' of about 5 days.

Sperm testing kits are also available. However, doctors do not recommend these because they cannot give the same level of accuracy or detail as a laboratory test.

Ovarian reserve testing (see below) has also given rise to home tests. These must be done in the first few days of the menstrual cycle. The simplest is a urine test strip to measure FSH. This is not recommended because the results need to be interpreted carefully and could be misleading. It is also possible to take a blood sample and send it off by post to a commercial laboratory, which will send your results with an explanation. Again, most doctors do not recommend this.

It is important to remember that positive results from home tests do not prove that you are fertile. Other factors such as blocked tubes could still cause infertility. If you have difficulty conceiving, it is best to get medical advice.

Fertility tests for the man

Semen analysis

You will be asked to provide a semen sample. The laboratory will have a special room where you can produce a sample in privacy, or you may prefer to bring it in from home. You should wait for about 3 days after the last ejaculation before the test.

The sample of semen for analysis should be produced by masturbation into a sterile container. The clinic will provide a sterile jar with a lid. Do not use withdrawal, as some sperm may be lost, or a condom, as this is coated with a chemical that will kill the sperm. If you are only able to produce the sample by having intercourse, ask the laboratory staff to provide a condom that does not affect the sperm.

The sample needs to reach the laboratory quickly—within an hour if possible, and at most 2 hours. If it is delayed, the vitality of the sperm will be lost, particularly if they get cold. Keep the jar close to body temperature by putting it in a trouser pocket or inside your jacket. Do not put it in the fridge!

The laboratory will measure the quantity of semen, check the appearance, and use a microscope to examine it. They will count the number of sperm in the sample and the proportion that are moving. They will also look at individual sperm to see if they have a normal shape and appearance. The laboratory may also test the sample for infection and antibodies (see Chapter 10).

Normal results are given in Chapter 10. If the results are not good, you will be asked to give another sample after a few weeks. Sperm counts can vary from time to time even in healthy men, and may be affected by recent events such as a virus infection, and so it is more reliable to look at two or more samples.

Further tests

If the sperm count is very low or there are no sperm at all, you will need further tests. A blood test can check your hormone levels and look for a genetic cause. A small operation may be advised to look for any blockage in the tubes carrying the sperm. A biopsy (a small piece of tissue) may be taken from the testis to see whether sperm are being produced.

Fertility tests for the woman

Are eggs being released? Tests of ovulation

A blood test for the hormone progesterone will show whether ovulation has occurred. Progesterone is only produced after ovulation (see Chapter 3). To get the best result, the blood sample must be taken mid-way between ovulation and the next period. Progesterone reaches a peak a week after ovulation, which is a week before the period is expected. This can be timed with urine testing, or calculated from the monthly cycle (for example, it is day 21 of a 28-day cycle). Urine tests for the hormone LH are described above in the section on home testing.

Ultrasound scanning can also be used to monitor the monthly cycle and show the development and release of the egg.

 Case study

Sameena had been married for more than a year when she went to her GP for help in getting pregnant. She was asked to have a blood test on day 21 of her cycle. When she went back, she was told that the result was poor and she was probably not ovulating. Sameena explained that her periods were not always regular; in fact, in the month she had the test, it was a week late. The GP explained how Sameena could chart her monthly cycle, and she bought a kit from the chemist to test her urine at home. She used up the whole box of test strips, but it gave a positive result on day 20, and a week later her GP repeated the blood test which confirmed that she was ovulating.

Are the ovaries working well? Ovarian reserve testing

Not every egg is a good one, and as women get older, they have fewer eggs in their ovaries and the quality of the eggs declines. The store of eggs in the ovaries is sometimes called the 'ovarian reserve'. Even some young women have low reserves. Testing for this is important because ovarian reserve predicts the woman's response to fertility drugs, and her chances of successful treatment.

Testing for ovarian reserve is done in the early days of the menstrual cycle, usually on day 3. At this stage the ovaries are quiet, and the hormones are at steady levels.

Ultrasound scanning will show the size of the ovaries. The number of visible egg sacs ('follicles') is a guide to the number of eggs stored in reserve. This is called the 'antral follicle count' (Figure 7.3). The hormone FSH, and sometimes oestradiol, AMH, or inhibin-B are measured using a blood test. FSH drives the ovaries to produce eggs (see Chapter 3). If they are working well, not much FSH is needed—a low FSH result is good. If the ovaries are struggling to produce eggs, FSH is driving them hard and its level rises—a high result is bad. Measuring more hormones may improve the accuracy of the test, but the use of oestradiol, AMH, and inhibin-B varies between clinics.

Can the eggs and sperm meet?

The sperm have a difficult journey through the cervix, through the womb, and into the Fallopian tubes to meet the egg (see Chapter 3). Meanwhile the egg is released from the ovary and has to be picked up by the Fallopian tube and

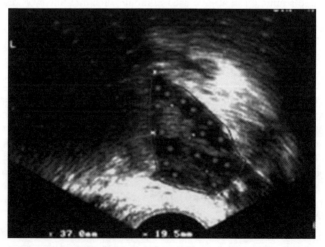

Figure 7.3 Ultrasound scan of ovary showing antral follicles.

carried down to the womb. Testing this passageway may involve ultrasound, X-rays, or minor surgery.

- Ultrasound scanning may show problems such as fibroids filling the cavity of the womb, or a blocked and swollen Fallopian tube.

- HyCoSy is an ultrasound test, which injects fluid into the womb so that it can pass upwards into the tubes where it is visible on scan.

- HSG is an X-ray of the womb and tubes. Fluid is injected through the cervix so that it outlines the cavity of the womb and passes upwards through the tubes. X-ray pictures are taken at the same time.

- Laparoscopy, often called 'lap and dye' is a minor operation. A telescope is passed through the navel to look inside the abdomen. This gives a clear view of the surface of the womb, tubes, and ovaries. Fluid is passed through the cervix and should be seen spilling out through the tubes inside the body. The fluid is tinted blue so that it can be seen easily, hence the name 'dye test'.

- Hysteroscopy is often done at the same time as laparoscopy—a tiny telescope is passed through the vagina and cervix to look inside the womb.

An ultrasound scan is often done first, as it is simple and painless. However, to make sure that the tubes are open, the most common test is an HSG X-ray. If a problem with the tubes is suspected, a laparoscopy will be recommended.

Ultrasound

This test uses sound waves which bounce off internal organs to create pictures. The scan probe (like a microphone) is put inside the vagina or on the lower part of your abdomen. The black-and-white pictures are seen on a screen and can be stored or printed (Figures 7.4 and 7.5). Ultrasound is simple, painless, and safe. It has been used for many years, and has never been shown to cause any ill effects.

HSG

An outpatient appointment will be made with the X-ray department shortly after your period has finished. You will be asked to undress and lie on the X-ray couch, and the doctor will do an internal examination (rather like having a cervical smear test). You may feel some discomfort, like period pains, as the fluid is injected. The test only takes a few minutes. The pictures are seen in black-and-white on a screen, and can be stored or printed (Figure 7.6).

You may be asked to take antibiotic cover for the HSG, as there is a small risk that germs from the cervix could be pushed upwards and cause infection. This is rare. You will be asked to avoid sex for a few days in case of infection. The X-ray itself will not cause damage, although it is very important that you are not pregnant at the time of the test—it is usually done early in the cycle once the period has finished but before ovulation (day 8 or 9).

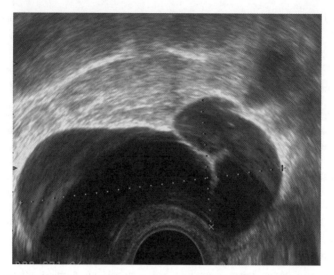

Figure 7.4 Ultrasound scan showing swollen tube ('hydrosalpinx'; see Chapter 22).

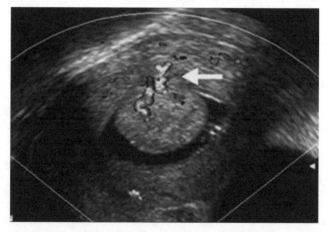

Figure 7.5 Ultrasound scan during HyCoSy, showing fibroid growing into the cavity of the womb. The fibroid is clearly outlined by fluid. The arrow shows the blood vessel feeding the fibroid.

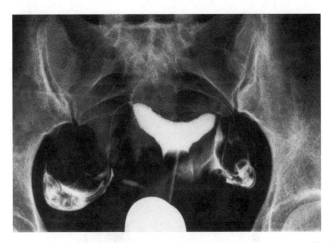

Figure 7.6 X-ray picture of HSG. The fluid shows up white in this picture as it fills the inside of the womb and both tubes, which are patent.

HSG is simple and quick, and it is the most common test for the tubes. It also gives useful views of the cavity inside the womb. HSG can occasionally give false results, for example if the tube goes into spasm it may appear blocked. If HSG shows a blockage, it is usually followed up by laparoscopy.

Laparoscopy

This is a small operation done under general anaesthetic, usually as a day case (without staying the night). You will be asked to come into hospital prepared for the anaesthetic by having had nothing to eat or drink for several hours beforehand. Once you are asleep, a small cut is made inside the navel and a telescope is put into the abdomen (Figure 7.7). To give space for the telescope, carbon dioxide gas (which is part of the air we breathe) is passed into the abdomen. A second small instrument is usually put in the lower abdomen to move the internal organs and lift the tubes to see them closely. Meanwhile, fluid is injected through the vagina and cervix, and can be seen spilling out through the tubes inside the body. Pictures are shown in colour on a screen and can be stored and printed (Figure 7.8). At the end of the operation, the instruments are removed and the gas is released. The cuts are closed with a couple of stitches or plaster strips.

You will probably be ready to go home about 4 hours after the laparoscopy. You should not go home alone, or try to drive for 24 hours after the anaesthetic. After a day or two resting at home you can go back to work. You will be advised not to have sex for a few days as there could be a risk of infection, and you may be asked to take a course of antibiotics.

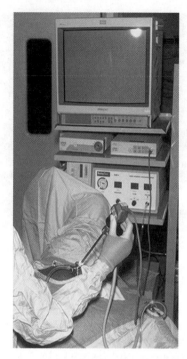

Figure 7.7 A laparoscopy operation, showing the telescope connected to a colour monitor.

The risk of complications from a laparoscopy is estimated as 1 in 300. The most serious risk is damage to the internal organs when the telescope is inserted. This could involve the bowel or blood vessels, and end up in a repair operation. A few deaths have occurred from laparoscopy. However, the risk is very small indeed for healthy women having infertility tests.

Laparoscopy is a much more invasive procedure than HSG, but it is more accurate and gives more information. It is used when tubal damage is suspected. It is also the best choice if you have a high chance of endometriosis (see Chapter 21), as this may not be detected by any other test.

Another advantage of laparoscopy is that it can be used to treat scarring (adhesions) and endometriosis. Some fertility specialists will offer this at the same time; they will look and see what the problem is, and then go on to treat it under the same anaesthetic. This means a bigger operation and longer stay in hospital, but recovery from keyhole surgery is quick, and hopefully you can become pregnant soon afterwards.

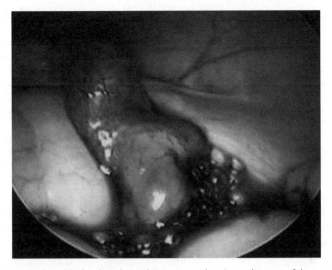

Figure 7.8 A photograph taken during laparoscopy, showing a close-up of the open end of the Fallopian tube with blue dye spilling through it.

Hysteroscopy

A very small telescope is put through the vagina and cervix to see inside the womb. Fluid or gas is passed along the telescope into the womb, stretching it open to give clear views. This is often combined with laparoscopy. It can also be done alone, either as an outpatient procedure or under general anaesthesia. It is used to investigate abnormal bleeding, to see fibroids or polyps, and to check the shape of the womb.

The risk of complications from hysteroscopy is very small indeed. The instrument could damage the womb, but this is rare and usually heals without a problem.

Hysteroscopy can also be used to remove fibroids or polyps, and take samples from the womb lining (it is the modern version of 'D&C').

Infection screening

Chlamydia is a common sexually transmitted disease, which may give no symptoms. Screening for Chlamydia is recommended for women before fertility tests and treatment. This can be done by a swab test or a urine test. If Chlamydia is present in the woman's cervix, there is a risk that the infection could be carried up into the tubes.

Testing for HIV, hepatitis B, and hepatitis C before starting fertility treatment is routine in the UK. These infections are becoming more common, and people may not be aware that they are infected. These viruses can be passed to other people in body fluids and through sexual intercourse, and also to a baby at delivery. Special precautions can be taken to reduce this risk, for example vaccination against hepatitis B is advised for sexual partners and for babies soon after birth. It is also important for any laboratory to be aware if they are handling blood or semen samples that could be infectious.

Testing for CMV (cytomegalovirus) is also recommended for sperm and egg donors and women being treated with donor gametes. CMV is a virus that causes a flu-like illness, not serious in itself, but carrying a risk of infecting an unborn baby. If a woman is not immune, there is a theoretical risk of catching CMV from donor sperm or eggs.

Pre-pregnancy checks for women

As explained in Chapter 2 (Preparing for pregnancy), it is sensible to check that you are immune to rubella (also called German measles). Catching rubella in pregnancy may cause severe damage to the developing baby, and can be prevented by vaccination.

There are a few inherited diseases that can be predicted by testing before pregnancy. Sickle cell disease is a good example. This is a blood disorder that is carried by many people of African descent. Carrying it is called 'sickle cell trait' and is not harmful, but if both the man and the woman carry it, there is a 1 in 4 chance that their child will inherit a double dose, causing serious illness. Other examples are thalassaemia in people of Mediterranean or South Asian descent, and Tay–Sachs disease in some Jewish families. Most fertility clinics will offer tests for these disorders.

Results of fertility tests

Try to see an experienced doctor or nurse to go through the results of your tests. It is important that they are explained in a way that you can understand. Results are not always 'good' or 'bad'—sometimes they are in between, and deciding whether to act on them can be difficult.

Look at the whole picture in deciding what to do next. Put the test results in context—how long you have been trying, and the woman's age, are also important in deciding on treatment.

If you are moving to another clinic for treatment, it is a good idea to get copies of your results. Take them with you to your appointment. This will give your specialists the information they need, and you will avoid repeating any tests unnecessarily.

8

Counselling: dealing with the emotional aspects of infertility

> **Key points**
>
> ◆ People often describe the experience of fertility treatment as an emotional roller coaster ride.
>
> ◆ The HFEA requires licensed clinics to offer counselling in appropriate surroundings by qualified counsellors.
>
> ◆ Counselling can be supportive, to help people deal with emotions like grief and anxiety.
>
> ◆ Therapeutic counselling might be suggested to help people whose infertility has caused old problems to resurface.
>
> ◆ Implications counselling is offered and sometimes insisted upon by the clinic to ensure that people are giving informed consent, particularly when using egg or sperm donation.

That roller coaster

By now you will probably have heard the expression 'roller coaster of emotions' a hundred times and may have experienced it as well. Whilst it is over-used, the image well describes two kinds of experience of fertility treatment. First, the highs and the lows: a good blood test result being followed by the arrival of a period, for example. Secondly, the sense of not being in control of your life any more but being swept along on some nightmare ride at the mercy of hormone levels, staff holidays, egg quality, sperm numbers, cysts, scans...

Having some time talking to a counsellor, who will have heard the experiences of many others, and putting words to your experiences can help you make sense of what is happening, feel less isolated, and assist in giving you back some sense of control.

Why have counselling? A little history

Counselling has to be offered in all licensed units. These are generally the clinics offering IVF which have to be inspected and licensed by the HFEA (see Chapter 5). This situation is unusual. The law does not require counselling to be offered anywhere else in the health system.

Louise Brown, the first IVF baby, was born in 1978, and now, 30 years later, it may seem surprising that there was a real fear that this new procedure could lead to all sorts of unacceptable scientific experiments and that people who were having difficulty getting pregnant might be tempted to try anything to have a child.

Counselling was really put in place to ensure that those in this particularly vulnerable situation had to be offered the time and attention with a fully qualified professional to think about what was going on and its implications. It was put there to help normal healthy adults deal with unusual and highly stressful situations. In the latest HFEA Code of Practice 2007 the requirement to offer counselling remains.

Why not have counselling?

If you have never even contemplated counselling before or have just had enough of sharing with yet another stranger all the most private details of your life, you may well decline the offer. Some people feel that it is only for those who 'aren't coping' and that whereas they have to allow the doctors to carry out the medical procedures to help them have a baby, talking to some kindly (usually) woman isn't going to make any difference.

You don't have to have counselling, but every unit needs to make sure that they help you to feel that counselling is an integral part of the treatment, not specially tacked on only for women who cry (which is, anyway, a very healthy response to bad news).

What is support counselling?

The HFEA Code of Practice requires three types of counselling to be offered. The most obvious one is called 'support counselling', which really 'does what it says on the tin'. It offers you support, if you want it, from someone with specialist knowledge of the impact of fertility problems on an individual or couple.

For instance, many people are ashamed, upset, and self-critical when they feel angry, resentful, or even just less loving towards friends or relatives who become pregnant. Sometimes they cannot visit anyone with a new baby for quite a long time, until the child is no longer 'a baby'. The counsellor can help you understand how normal and expected this kind of reaction can be, and that you are not a horrible person to feel this—just you, in a horrible situation, and that you might be feeling envious of the person with the baby, something you probably haven't experienced for many years. Normally in adult life, if you want something, you'll strive to get it: the job; the partner; somewhere to live; the holiday; the qualification; that gadget; that dress. You'll save money, plan, or you might decide that you don't really want it that much, or can't afford it, but in all these things there is an element of control and choice. When you plan to have a baby, as friends and relatives are doing, and it doesn't happen, you have to hand yourself over to 'experts' who seem to be doing things on your behalf that are not working for the two of you on your own. They put the egg and the sperm together, not you and your partner in a loving sex act. The most intimate aspects of bodies and lives are investigated and chronicled, and you wait to be told what is going to happen to you, what can be done or not done for you. The only choice you can make is to stop—that is your only bit of control and it is unthinkable because this is not depriving yourself of a holiday, it's depriving you of the future you have grown up believing in. Wanting to create your own family is part of your identity.

This can be a life crisis, so maybe needing counselling support that you would never normally have contemplated is not such an unthinkable step.

The counselling session

The counselling should take place in a quiet dedicated space for about 50 minutes, so that it is not rushed or interrupted. You should have issues of confidentiality explained to you. Very rarely, if the counsellor thinks that you might be at serious risk of harming yourself or somebody else or any children, or potential children might be at risk, they would have to tell you that this information needs to be shared with the clinic team.

Time for you

The session will really be your space to use as you want to, to have a good moan, argue, discuss with your partner, cry, complain, and explore with a professional 'listener' what it feels like to be *you* going through this process. The counsellor (who is also inspected by the HFEA) will listen and learn from you. He/she will respond without making any judgements, will acknowledge what you are telling them, and try to show you how your responses, which might seem bizarre to you, are in fact quite usual for people in your stressful situation.

Time for reflection

The counsellor might also help put into words some of the thoughts and feelings that you haven't been able to talk about to anybody else. For example, some women realize that they are even jealous of their own mother because, of course, she has had a daughter. Some mothers aren't very helpful, bemoaning the absence of grandchildren, and the counsellor would be able to put into words feelings of anger towards the mother, which are in fact not uncommon but might feel like a betrayal to the woman concerned. The counsellor might reflect back what has been said to make sure that you feel you have been understood, and might link up various issues that could clarify particular areas of difficulty—for instance, that a couple always seem to have an argument after visiting friends with children.

The counsellor, in the position of detached but caring observer, may help the couple make the connection that they are too close and involved to be able to discern.

Therapeutic counselling

Painful memories

For some people, the experience of dealing with infertility may trigger memories of painful personal struggles in the past or other deeper longer-lasting psychological difficulties.

For instance, if you were adopted, or had lost a parent at a young age your need to create your own genetic family or become a mother to your own child might feel particularly desperate. Maybe you have suffered from depression or mental health problems, and the stress and uncertainty of what you are going through now might be a real struggle.

Relationship difficulties

Your relationship with your partner may be in difficulties. Sex, which would previously have been a source of pleasure and togetherness, may well have become a timed chore and feel pointless because it hasn't worked.

You are not being judged

Counselling in these circumstances should really offer support, in that it is non-judgemental, empathic, culturally aware, and easily available, but should also be able to offer you the possibility of exploring older problems that predated the fertility problems but are impacting on how you are able to cope with these.

The counsellor attached to the clinic may be able to offer therapeutic counselling or advise and assist you to see someone else. This might be someone who specializes in couple counselling or sexual problems, perhaps a long-term psychotherapist or a specialist in cognitive–behaviour therapy, which can be very helpful if you are prone to anxiety or phobias. Unfortunately, these sessions will almost undoubtedly have to be paid for, and many private units also charge for support counselling. However, when old unresolved problems affect the way you cope with current difficulties, this kind of intervention could be really helpful.

Implications counselling

This is rather a different form of counselling and is really more of a discussion between you and the counsellor to ensure that you will be giving 'informed consent'. It is an extension of the conversation you will have had with your clinician, with more social, psychological, and emotional topics to consider.

You may well have an implications counselling session if you are using your own sperm and eggs. In these sessions you might be asked to think about the risks of multiple pregnancies, how any child from this treatment might affect other children already in your family, what you want to do with surplus embryos, and what instructions you would leave if you died and had frozen embryos. This is not a test with right or wrong answers, just a sort of checklist to make sure you have thought of some of the many different aspects of fertility treatment.

Treatment involving donors and surrogacy

Implications counselling should always be offered and sometimes insisted upon when you need to use donor eggs, sperm, or embryos. If you need surrogacy, there will certainly be a requirement for both you and your surrogate to have counselling.

It has to be very clear that this counselling session is *not* a form of assessment, because it often seems to be experienced like that by many people. As you probably know, the law has changed and any donor-conceived child now has the right, when they are 18, to know the identity of their donor (if the treatment has taken place in the UK) and, after receiving counselling, they have a right to make contact. As you also are probably very aware, this has resulted in a shortage of donors at present.

What should you tell your child?

If you are using donor sperm, eggs, or embryos, you will be asked to think about whether you feel you should tell a child. The counsellor will be able to help you with information and advice if you feel that it is important not to have such a big secret kept at the heart of your family. If you don't plan to tell (in which case any child would also not know about their right to know who their donor was), you will be asked to think about the problems of unplanned disclosure and how that might be managed. You will be asked to consider what it would feel like to carry a child who is not genetically yours, or how you feel about your partner having another man's sperm put inside them.

If you are using a known donor (a friend or a relative), the counsellor will point out that if, for instance, you were using your sister's eggs, your child would be both cousin and half-sibling to her children and ask you all to consider how best this should be dealt with. You will need to think about what would happen if either or both of you died and you had stored sperm, eggs, or embryos. You will need to know that until the embryo is put back inside the woman, the donor has rights over the embryo and could refuse permission for its use.

This may all sound rather brutal, but it is really to help you face 'nitty-gritty' issues which might not have occurred to you while there is still time to have discussions about what you want to do, or to change your mind before it's too late if you find some of the implications unacceptable.

Donors will also be offered implications counselling and of course they too might change their minds, which can be very painful for the potential recipients. This is just the sort of experience which brings you back to the roller coaster and how counselling might feel like a hand to hold on the miserable descent as well as on the long slow climb to the top.

9

Complementary and alternative medicine (CAM)

> ## ➜ Key points
>
> ◆ Complementary and alternative medicine (CAM) may be useful for couples where traditional investigations have not identified the reason for the delay in getting pregnant or for those who want to try alternatives to conventional approaches.
>
> ◆ CAM treatments can also be more attractive as they tend to be less invasive than conventional methods.
>
> ◆ Commonly used CAM treatments include acupuncture, traditional Chinese medicine (TCM), hair analysis, osteopathy, reflexology, and reiki.

Traditional medicine examines the disease process and treats disease. Practitioners of CAM view the body and mind as a whole and believe that stress plays a major role in contributing to health problems, including difficulty in getting pregnant. Patients may seek out CAM clinicians to provide explanations for the cause of symptoms, often when conventional medicine has been unable to do so.

Many of us have friends who have become pregnant after CAM treatment, but there is little 'scientific evidence' to prove that CAM is effective. Lack of funding, lack of a research mindset, and difficulty in testing CAM treatments are the major problems limiting research.

CAM treatments may be useful for couples where traditional investigations have not identified a reason for their delay in getting pregnant and so have been advised to continue trying for a while longer before starting fertility treatment.

Another group are those who have reached the end of the line in terms of fertility treatment and want to try alternatives. CAM approaches may also be attractive as they generally tend to be less invasive.

Many CAM practitioners believe that nutrition is important and will address any vitamin and trace element deficiencies, particularly zinc, magnesium, and omega 3.

As with traditionally trained doctors, not all CAM practitioners are experienced in treating fertility problems. Before embarking on a course of treatment with any particular practitioner it would be sensible to enquire about their fertility-related experience.

Acupuncture and traditional Chinese medicine

Traditional Chinese medicine (TCM) originated in China over 2000 years ago. It teaches that the body relies on the qi (sometimes written as chi) or 'vital energy' to remain healthy (analogous to reiki—see below). The flow of the qi can be blocked by an imbalance of two opposing forces, the ying and the yang. When this happens, a disease process can result. Thus the ying and the yang should be re-balanced to restore good health.

The qi flows around the body along meridians or pathways: there are 12 main meridians and eight secondary ones. The ying–yang balance can be restored by various methods according to TCM: herbs may be prescribed, or massage and meditation may be used. Acupuncture can affect qi by connecting with the meridians via identified acupuncture points, of which there are over 2000 on the body. These points can be stimulated in a variety of ways, the most common being with a very fine needle the width of a hair. If you are considering acupuncture, you should ensure that your acupuncturist only uses single-use sterile needles to reduce any possibility of introducing infection.

Of all forms of CAM, acupuncture is probably the one that has been subjected to the most research. Certainly there is good evidence that it can reduce the nausea and vomiting caused by chemotherapy and can also reduce pain. However, its effect is still not understood. It may be able to alter the release of the body's natural painkillers and possibly affect the immune system, blood pressure, and blood flow.

There have been several scientific studies of the effects of acupuncture on fertility or fertility treatment. Although most (but not all) have shown a possible benefit, the number of subjects recruited into the trials is generally small and the demonstrated positive effect is minimal. In addition, not all the studies have excluded the 'placebo effect' of treatment.

Hair analysis

Hair analysis has become popular as a method of detecting nutritional deficiencies. Although hair analysis can be used to detect exposure to certain poisons and heavy metals (e.g. lead, mercury, and arsenic), there is no evidence that it can predict nutritional problems.

Osteopathy

Osteopathy was the first CAM profession to achieve an Act of Parliament in the UK. The Osteopaths Act was passed in 1993 and all UK osteopaths are now statutorily regulated and follow strict codes of professional practice and ethics.

Biomechanical function includes that of the nerves, muscles, and skeleton, usually means alteration in range and quality of movement and changes in tissue texture quality. A good example of biomechanical dysfunction is low back pain. Osteopaths have become recognized as experts in musculoskeletal pain syndromes such as low back pain, and are often able to identify relevant disturbances in biomechanical function. Symptoms may improve with the appropriate osteopathic treatment. The internal organs may develop analogous biomechanical problems which contribute to difficulties in getting pregnant. Improvement in biomechanical function may improve the nerve supply and blood supply to the pelvic reproductive organs, a central tenet of osteopathic philosophy. Theoretically this could improve reproductive function.

Osteopaths believe that head and neck techniques improve hypothalamic–pituitary function (and therefore the hormones that control the reproductive organs) and back techniques improve adrenal function (again important in the production of hormones, particularly those involved in stress). Many osteopathic techniques dampen down the effects of stress on the body. Exercises such as Pilates, yoga, and tai chi are often recommended by osteopaths to counteract the effects of stress.

Reflexology

In reflexology it is believed that the different internal and external parts of the body are represented on the feet and the hands. By applying pressure to the relevant part of the foot or hand, the function of the corresponding organ can be affected. Most people describe feeling relaxed and stress free after reflexology, although there is no direct evidence that it works other than as a relaxation technique.

Reiki

Reiki is a form of hands-on healing, originating in Japan, which takes its name from the word meaning 'universal energy'. It is believed to harness the same energy as acupuncture, tai chi, and yoga. Practitioners use reiki to treat a variety of physical, emotional, relationship, and stress-related problems. A typical treatment involves the client lying fully clothed on a massage couch while the practitioner places his/her hands over the body. Some people even describe a tingling sensation or one of warmth during or after a session.

Couples trying for a baby often experience high levels of stress, particularly if medical intervention is required. The longer it takes, of course, the more anxious they become and the more chance there is of stress inhibiting fertility. Long work hours can have a similar detrimental effect on fertility. Many patients do not recognize that stress may be affecting them. Most CAM treatments are pleasant to experience and there may well be a beneficial effect on fertility as an indirect result, probably by helping to relieve stress and to foster a more positive mental attitude.

10

Male fertility

 Key points

◆ Male fertility is the main problem in approximately one in three couples unable to get pregnant.

◆ There is no male 'biological clock', and men can theoretically continue fathering children into old age.

◆ Semen analysis can vary from day to day, and so it is important to repeat the test if the result is abnormal.

◆ Fertility drugs are not effective for men, but laboratory preparation of semen with assisted conception give good success rates.

It takes two to make a baby

It is just as important that the man attend the fertility appointment and is thoroughly checked over. It is estimated that male fertility is the main problem in one in three couples trying to get pregnant. Overall about 75 per cent of couples will conceive after trying for a year.

Unlike women, there is no male biological clock and men can theoretically continue fathering children into old age.

Sperm are produced in the testes and are stored in the epididymis to mature. It takes about 64 days to produce a mature sperm. About 100–200 million sperm are produced every day and this process continues throughout a man's life. Each sperm has a characteristic head with a nucleus which contains the male genetic material (Figure 10.1). There is a also a tail, which allows the sperm to swim inside the female partner.

When a man has an orgasm, ejaculatory fluid or semen is expelled from his penis (Figure 10.2). Less than 1 per cent of this fluid is made up of sperm. The rest consists of secretions from other glands, including the prostate and the seminal vesicles. This fluid contains chemicals, such as fructose and zinc, which are important for the normal functioning of sperm.

Approximately 40–80 million sperm are ejaculated and these sperm swim the equivalent of the Atlantic Ocean in order to reach the egg. At the end of this arduous journey, one of these sperm must burrow its way into the egg in order to achieve fertilization. Millions of sperm are produced so that the chances of a single sperm reaching an egg are increased.

Fertility is a question not just of sperm number but also of quality. The motility of the sperm is also important for fertilization to occur. A man may have a normal sperm count but if the sperm are not moving well pregnancy may not occur. This also applies to the number of normal forms. Humans can produce many abnormal forms. However, if there are too many, this will affect the fertilizing potential of the sperm.

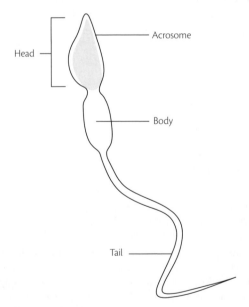

Figure 10.1 A spermatozoon/sperm.

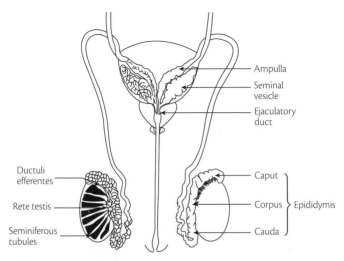

Figure 10.2 The passages of the male genital tract. Reproduced from Serhal, P., and Overton, O., (2004) *Good Clinical Practice in Assisted Reproduction*, pp. 226–55 and originally from Whitfield, H.N., Hendry, W.F., Kirby, R.S., and Duckett, J.W., (1998) *Textbook of Genitourinary Surgery*, 2nd edn, with permission of Wiley-Blackwell Publishing.

Male hormones

Testosterone is the main male hormonez and is produced by the testes. The production of testosterone and sperm begins at puberty. Follicle-stimulating hormone (FSH) and luteinizing hormone (LH) are produced by the pituitary gland in the brain and control sperm and testosterone production. Pituitary problems are rare, but can result in male fertility problems. If the testicles are damaged, the FSH and LH levels in the body rise in an effort to increase sperm and testosterone production.

Semen analysis can vary from day to day, and so it is important to repeat the test if the result is abnormal. It is also important to follow the instructions for producing the semen for analysis as the quality and quantity may change according to how the sample was produced. The first part of the ejaculate usually contains most of the moving sperm and is often the hardest to catch. If the semen analysis or the repeat is normal, further investigations will concentrate on the woman.

Instructions for production of a semen sample

◆ The sample should be produced by masturbation after 3–4 days of abstinence.

◆ The sample should be kept warm (in an inside pocket of a jacket) and should be delivered to the laboratory for analysis as soon as possible (and no longer than 2 hours after production). If you live too far away to do this, it may be possible to produce the sample at the fertility clinic in a private room reserved for this purpose.

◆ The first part of the ejaculate contains most of the moving sperm. It is important to try and catch the entire sample in the bottle provided.

◆ The process of sperm production takes 3 months, so sperm quality can be affected by recent ill health. Therefore it is normal practice to repeat the semen analysis if the first sample shows a low value.

> **Fact:** The sample cannot be collected into a condom as the spermicide and chemicals in the condom affect sperm quality. It should not be refrigerated as the sperm will die at low temperatures.

Semen analysis

Sperm can be seen under the microscope wiggling their tails which moves them forwards. This movement, which is called progressive motility, is thought to be very important for fertilization of the egg, where the sperm has to burrow through the egg wall. Some sperm can be seen to swim round and round in circles, or simply shake on the spot. The motility of the sperm is graded according to certain criteria. Normally more than 50 per cent of the sperm should be moving with good progression. Humans produce large numbers of abnormal forms or shapes. It is possible to have up to 85 per cent abnormal forms and still be fertile.

More detailed analysis such as the mixed antiglobulin reaction (MAR test) for sperm antibodies can be done at the same time, although is not performed at all laboratories.

Normal semen analysis

◆ Volume greater than 2 ml

◆ Total sperm number more than 40 million

◆ Sperm concentration more than 20 million sperm per millilitre

◆ Motility more than 50 per cent with progressive motion or more than 25 per cent with rapid progressive motion

◆ More than 15 per cent of the sperm have a normal shape

◆ Less than 1 million white cells per millilitre (more than this may indicate an infection)

Post-coital test

This test is no longer commonly done. The post-coital test is predictive of pregnancy where fertility is unexplained and the couple have been trying for less than 3 years. Couples with a negative post-coital test should move to assisted fertility treatment sooner, and those with a positive result have a good chance of natural conception if they continue trying.

Cervical mucus is a barrier that must be crossed by sperm on their journey to fertilize the egg. The post-coital test assesses the sperm–mucus interaction. The couple should have intercourse the night before the day of testing, which should be as close as possible to ovulation. The cervical mucus is examined under the microscope for the presence of progressively moving sperm.

> A positive post-coital test is one where there are progressively moving sperm in the cervical mucus.

Male fertility problems and treatment

A low volume of semen

This may be due to retrograde ejaculation where the sperm pass backwards into the bladder. This problem is common after prostate surgery and can occur in men with diabetes. Men with retrograde ejaculation can be treated with drugs such as ephedrine or imipramine. These drugs are thought to contract the bladder neck muscle, thus preventing semen passing into the bladder after ejaculation. About one in three men respond to treatment. Alternatively, sperm can be recovered from the urine and used for intra-uterine insemination (see Chapter 12) or IVF (see Chapter 14). If this fails, sperm can be retrieved directly from the testicle.

In men with anorgasmia (inability to ejaculate), electro-ejaculation using stimulation with a vibrator may be combined with intra-uterine insemination or IVF. Occasionally sperm retrieval is needed to obtain sperm directly from the testicle.

A low volume may also be due to a blockage in the ejaculatory ducts at the level of the prostate which may result in fewer secretions and so a reduction in the volume of ejaculate. Surgery may be successful in unblocking these tubes.

Causes of retrograde ejaculation

- Spinal cord problems
- Multiple sclerosis
- Diabetes mellitus
- Abdominal surgery
- Prostate surgery

Oligozoospermia

This means that there are too few sperm within the ejaculate. It is often associated with too many abnormal forms (teratozoospermia) or reduced numbers of motile sperm (asthenozoospermia). If all three are present, this is often termed OATS (oligo, astheno, teratozoospermia).

Up to one in four men will have no obvious cause for their abnormal result.

There are many causes of OATS and some of these are listed below:

- idiopathic or unknown
- undescended testicles
- varicoceles (varicose veins in the scrotum)
- drugs and chemicals
- chemotherapy
- radiotherapy
- genito-urinary infection
- hormone problems
- partial ejaculatory duct obstruction
- genetic causes.

Azoospermia

This term means that there are no sperm in the semen sample. This may be because there is a block in the tubes from the testes or because sperm are not being produced in sufficient quantity. Hormone tests will help to decide between the two explanations.

If sperm are being produced, the testes are usually of normal size and the level of the pituitary gland hormone (FSH) is normal. If sperm are not being produced sufficiently, the testes are usually small and the FSH level is high. This is often termed testicular failure and some of the causes are outlined in the box.

Causes of testicular failure

- Drugs and chemicals
- Radiotherapy
- Genetic
- Undescended testicles
- Trauma and infections
- Mumps

A chromosomal analysis should be carried out in men with extremely low sperm counts (less than 5 million sperm per millilitre) and men who are azoospermic.

Sometimes, men can be born with genetic problems which may cause the azoospermia. One of these is Klinefelter's syndrome, where the man carries an extra X chromosome.

The Y chromosome is important for producing sperm and recently it has been shown that men with both azoospermia and oligospermia may have deletions on their Y chromosomes which cause their fertility problem. The use of ICSI to treat men with Y chromosome deletions may result in an identical form of infertility in any male children born. Unfortunately, there is no treatment to correct a chromosomal abnormality.

Sperm, which can be used for ICSI, can be obtained in up to 50 per cent of men who have testicular failure or whose testicles are not working properly. A relatively new technique, called micro-dissection testicular exploration and sperm extraction, uses an operating microscope to try and find sperm.

Obstructive azoospermia

Sperm are being produced, but are not being released because either no tubes are present (congenital bilateral absence of the vas deferens) or they have been damaged and blocked by infection or surgery (e.g. hernia repair or operations to remove epididymal cysts).

If the tubes are absent, additional tests are required. One is a check of the kidneys. There is a link between this condition and an absent kidney or a pelvic kidney. The other is testing for the cystic fibrosis gene after proper discussion, as up to 70 per cent of men with congenital absence of the vas deferens will be carriers of the cystic fibrosis gene.

Causes of obstruction or blockages

- Congenital absence of the vas
- Congenital cysts
- Infections
- Trauma
- Surgery of the testicles or hernias

If sperm are not being produced because of a blockage, your doctor will look for the reason. This may involve surgery to unblock the tubes or in some cases sperm may simply be taken directly from the testicle and used for IVF treatment. If the problem isn't treatable, the options open to you are donor insemination (sperm donation) or adoption (see Chapters 11 and 25).

Drugs and chemicals can also reduce sperm production. You should check with your doctor to see if any medication you are taking can cause this problem. Stopping a particular medication may improve the sperm count. Some drugs need to be withdrawn slowly, so always check with your doctor first.

Substances which reduce the sperm count

Anabolic steroids	Colchicine
Alcohol	Opioids
Sulfasalazine	Antibiotics: nitrofurantoin, aminoglycosides
Steroids	Cyproterone acetate
Cannabis	Diethylstilboestriol
Anticonvulsants	Pesticides

Varicocele

Varicoceles are varicose veins of the testis. (There is a sensation of a 'bag of worms'). The theory is that the increased blood supply keeps the testis too warm and this affects sperm production. The majority of varicoceles do not require an operation. Medical opinions differ as to whether fixing a varicocele with an operation will affect fertility. The current thinking is that it will not increase pregnancy rates, although it may improve oligozoospermia. Up to 15 per cent of men who have fathered children will have a varicocele and this figure increases to 30 per cent of men with infertility.

Surgery should only be carried out for for men with reduced sperm counts (less than 20 million sperm per millilitre, reduced motility, and abnormal sperm morphology) with the hope of improving sperm quality. Sperm quality normally recovers between 3 months and a year after surgery. However, the varicocele can recur, and recurrence rates as high as one in three have been reported.

Varicocele surgery should be carried out through the abdomen (tummy) rather than the scrotum, either laparoscopically or as a traditional open operation. More recently, a microsurgical operation has been described, with reported lower recurrence rates. Complications of surgical varicocele repair are hydrocele (increased fluid around the testis), damage to the testicular artery causing further deterioration in sperm production, and reappearance of the varicocele.

Undescended testis

Undescended testis in childhood may be a cause of infertility in some men. If the testis is not in the scrotum by 1 year of age, irreversible damage to the sperm-producing cells can occur. Occasionally it is possible to retrieve sperm from an undescended testis.

Hormone problems

Hormone problems in men are rare. Men with an underactive pituitary can often be successfully treated with hormones (human chorionic gonadotrophin HCG) or a combination of HCG and human menopausal gonadotrophin (HMG).

Idiopathic or unexplained male factor fertility

There is little evidence that fertility drug treatment works for male fertility problems. In the UK, fertility drugs are not recognized as treatment for unexplained male infertility.

A number of agents have been tried, including anti-oestrogens, androgens, and bromocriptine. There is some evidence that anti-oestrogens improve sperm quality, but no evidence that this is reflected in increased pregnancy rates. Similarly, treatment with androgens remains controversial and in fact in high doses they can be harmful to sperm production.

A number of studies suggest that treatment with anti-oxidants, mast cell blockers, and alpha-blockers improve sperm quality (and pregnancy rates) in men with low sperm counts (oligospermia) or no sperm counts (azoospermia). The place of steroids in treatment is controversial and they are not recommended. Some studies have reported improved pregnancy rates for men treated with anti-sperm antibodies, but significant side effects are associated with taking long-term steroids.

Fertility treatment for specific male fertility problems

Sperm can be obtained from the testis by a variety of techniques and can then be used for IVF/ICSI treatment. Sperm that is not immediately being used for

IVF/ICSI can be frozen. In practice, it is difficult to coordinate sperm extraction and egg collection on the same day, and sperm extraction is usually carried out before the IVF/ICSI cycle to be certain that sperm can be retrieved.

Sperm retrieval techniques (PESA, MESA, TESE)

There are a number of different types of technique for retrieving sperm for ICSI. The choice will depend upon the cause of the fertility problem.

Percutaneous epididymal aspiration of sperm (PESA)

Sperm can be recovered from the epididymis as an alternative to reversal of vasectomy (see Chapter 21), in cases of obstruction, or in congenital absence of the vas deferens. Under local anaesthetic, a needle is passed through the skin of the scrotum into the epididymis and sperm are retrieved. There are few complications and the procedure is not too uncomfortable. Sometimes the procedure needs to be carried out under a general anaesthetic; this depends upon how easy it is to feel the sperm tubes. Sometimes sperm cannot be retrieved from the epididymis or testicle under local anaesthetic and a cut needs to be made on the testicle under a general anaesthetic.

Micro-epididymal sperm aspiration (MESA)

Sperm is recovered from the epididymis during an operation (e.g. reversal of vasectomy). A microscope identifies a tube within the epididymis and a cut is made directly into this tube to recover sperm.

Testicular sperm extraction (TESE)

It is possible to recover sperm directly from the testis. This is done when there is testicular failure or sperm are not recoverable because of obstruction in the epididymis.

Sperm can be retrieved from the testicle by inserting a needle and extracting sperm (TESE), multiple biopsies where a cut is made on the testicle and wide areas of the testis are sampled, or a microdissection operation where an operating microscope is used to retrieve sperm after making a cut on the testicle. The sperm retrieval rates are higher using the microdissection technique than using the other techniques.

The pregnancy rates with epididymal sperm or testicular sperm for IVF/ICSI are similar, although this is controversial. The fertilization and pregnancy rates for ICSI using cryopreserved or fresh sperm are also similar.

11

Treatment options before IVF

Key points

◆ The reason for infertility can be pinpointed for many couples.

◆ 'Unexplained infertility' is diagnosed when tests have excluded all the major causes of infertility. It is quite common, and can affect up to 25 per cent of couples.

◆ The main treatment options given before IVF include intra-uterine insemination (IUI), superovulation, and superovulation combined with IUI.

◆ IUI is a simple treatment carried out in an outpatient clinic. It is often used to overcome mild male infertility, infertility associated with mild endometriosis, and unexplained infertility.

◆ Superovulation, or 'controlled ovarian hyperstimulation', involves the administration of fertility drugs (e.g. clomifene citrate or gonadotrophin injection) with the aim of releasing more than one egg.

◆ Success rates of treatment are higher if superovulation is combined with IUI.

The publicity given to IVF in magazines and television programmes gives the impression that IVF is the only form of fertility treatment. However, many couples can become pregnant with simpler treatment. A good clinic will investigate each couple carefully and give advice according to their individual circumstances. In general, it is best to start with the simplest effective treatment, and if this does not succeed, to proceed to the more complex techniques of IVF.

Treating the cause of infertility

The reason for infertility can be pinpointed for many couples. For example, if the woman has very infrequent periods and is not ovulating because she has polycystic ovaries, treatment to stimulate ovulation should be all that is necessary. Many men who want children after vasectomy will be best treated with an operation to reverse the vasectomy. See Chapter 13 for ovulation induction, Chapter 22 for tubal surgery, Chapter 21 for surgical treatment of endometriosis, and Chapter 23 for reversal of sterilization and reversal of vasectomy.

What if no cause is found?

'Unexplained infertility' is quite common. It is diagnosed when tests have excluded all the major causes of infertility. Semen analysis is normal, ovulation is confirmed, and the Fallopian tubes are open. This happens in up to one in four infertile couples. In some of these couples a subtle problem may be found on further testing; for example, laparoscopy may show fine adhesions even though HSG showed open tubes, or egg quality may be poor even though ovulation occurs regularly. A practical approach to 'unexplained infertility' is described below.

Wait and see

If no cause for fertility problems can be identified, there is no obvious barrier to conception and the outlook for a natural pregnancy may be good. It depends upon the age of the woman and the length of time the couple have been trying.

For example, if a couple have been trying for a year and the woman is aged under 30, there is at least a 50:50 chance of conceiving during the next year. It may be best for them to do nothing—just wait and see for a while. On the other hand, if a couple have already been trying for 3 years, their chance of natural pregnancy is not high even if no cause is found. They should be offered treatment straight away, usually with superovulation and IUI (see below). If they have been trying for 5 years or more, they should usually go straight to IVF.

For women over 35, and especially over 38, the time in which treatment will be effective may be limited, so even if no problem is found, they should move on promptly to treatment. Over the age of 38, it may be best to consider IVF.

Intra-uterine insemination

Intra-uterine insemination is usually abbreviated to IUI. A semen sample is prepared in the laboratory to extract and concentrate the healthy sperm, resulting in a small volume of fluid (half a millilitre) containing fertile sperm, which is drawn up into a very fine tube and passed through the cervix (Figure 11.1). The sample is then released into the womb so that the sperm are flushed up the Fallopian tubes.

Intra-uterine insemination is a simple treatment which is carried out in the clinic at an outpatient visit. It is similar to having a cervical smear test; it only takes a few minutes, and does not need an anaesthetic. Sometimes the IUI is

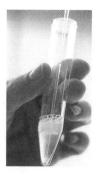

Figure 11.1 Preparation of sperm for IUI.

done with ultrasound guidance, and sometimes a full bladder may be needed. Most units advise a short rest before leaving the clinic.

To be effective, IUI has to be carried out on the day of ovulation or just before ovulation. This is timed using urine testing for the LH surge or HCG injection. Sometimes two inseminations are done on successive days. Usually the male partner's fresh sperm sample is used, and this needs to be produced on the day of treatment. It takes an hour or more to prepare the sample for IUI. Couples may be asked to abstain from sex for two or three days before the treatment, but it is fine to make love afterwards.

IUI is often used to overcome mild male infertility, when the sperm count is slightly low (but usually above 5 million moving sperm). Sperm washing for IUI can also remove anti-sperm antibodies. IUI can use donor sperm or the partner's stored frozen-thawed sperm (for example, if he has previously stored samples before cancer therapy).

IUI is often the first line of treatment for unexplained infertility. It is also used for infertility associated with mild endometriosis. IUI is also used for women whose infertility is believed to be due to cervical problems. For example, previous treatment for abnormal smear tests may have required a cone biopsy that has removed part of the cervix, reducing the production of cervical mucus.

Success rates from IUI will depend on the cause of infertility. They are usually around 10 per cent per cycle, but are higher with donor sperm and lower with endometriosis. It is such a simple treatment that it can be repeated in the next monthly cycle, and the chance of success accumulates over several months. Usually three to six treatments are carried out before moving on to IVF.

IUI carries very little risk of complications. Theoretically, infection could be carried into the womb during the procedure, but this is rare. Occasionally cramping pain can occur during the IUI procedure, particularly if the semen is not sufficiently washed. The chance of ectopic pregnancy (see Chapter 24) may be slightly raised.

Superovulation

Superovulation, or 'controlled ovarian hyperstimulation', means that fertility drugs are given with the aim of growing and releasing more than one egg. When given to a woman who is already ovulating naturally, these drugs boost her fertility and thus increase the chance of pregnancy.

The simplest, least invasive, and cheapest type of fertility drug is clomifene citrate. This is taken as a course of tablets for 5 days, starting early in the monthly cycle (usually on the third day of the period). In unexplained infertility, the chance of pregnancy is at least doubled by using clomifene. There is a risk of multiple birth; about one in ten pregnancies are twins, but triplets are very rare. The most common side effect of clomifene is hot flushes.

The other fertility drug used is gonadotrophin, which is given by injection. Several brands are available; they all contain FSH, which acts directly on the ovaries. A small dose is given daily or on alternate days, starting early in the menstrual cycle, usually by injection under the skin (similar to insulin injections for diabetes). The main risk of this treatment is multiple birth, and it can cause ovarian hyperstimulation (see Chapter 15).

Because of the risk of multiple pregnancy with this treatment, it is essential to monitor the cycle with ultrasound to check the number of eggs developing. Most cycles lead to the release of two or three eggs. This leads to higher success rates but all couples should be warned of the risk of multiple birth, which is usually around one in ten. If too many eggs develop, the treatment may be cancelled and resumed the next month. Alternatively, some couples may be offered 'follicle reduction' which removes excess eggs with ultrasound guidance, or the treatment cycle might be converted to IVF.

Superovulation and IUI

Success rates of treatment are higher if superovulation is combined with IUI. As a rule of thumb, this will treble the chance of pregnancy per cycle compared with trying naturally. Reported success rates range from 10 to 20 per cent per cycle (one in ten to one in five).

Superovulation and IUI is a very common treatment in the UK for unexplained infertility or mild fertility problems. Usually it is recommended for 3 or 4 months; if pregnancy has not been achieved, couples are then advised to consider IVF.

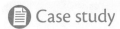 Case study

Rory and Janet were both schoolteachers, and had been married for 3 years when Janet stopped taking the Pill. They were expecting to get pregnant at once, but nothing happened for a year and they felt very frustrated when their doctor could not find any reason. Even worse, he suggested that they should wait another year before starting any treatment. They decided to go to a private clinic, and made an appointment for the school holidays. Just before their first visit, Janet's period had not occurred, and in fact she was pregnant naturally.

12

Problems with ovulation and polycystic ovary syndrome

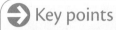 **Key points**

- Polycystic ovary syndrome (PCOS) is the most common hormone disorder in women of reproductive age, and is the most common cause of anovulation.

- 'Classic' symptoms of PCOS include lack of ovulation, irregular periods, hirsutism, and excessive acne.

- Other causes of anovulation include hypothalamic–pituitary failure, premature ovarian failure, and other hormone problems.

Anovulation means that you are either not releasing eggs (ovulating) or only releasing eggs sometimes. If you are not ovulating, periods are often irregular and there may be long gaps between them, perhaps lasting for 2 months or more. Alternatively, periods may occur more frequently than every 26 days. The period itself may be very light, perhaps little more than spotting of blood, lasting only a day or so. Another pattern sometimes seen is that the period may be very prolonged and last for more than 2 weeks.

Cycle length is counted as the number of days between the first day of one period and the first day of the next period (see Chapter 1). Periods are considered regular if, over a period of 6 months or more, the cycle varies by less than 5 days. You are likely to be ovulating regularly if your period cycle is regular.

Examples of a regular ovulatory cycle and an irregular anovulatory cycle are given in Boxes 12.1 and 12.2.

Box 12.1 A regular cycle

April

Sun	Mon	Tue	Wed	Thu	Fri	Sat
①	2	3	4	5	6	
7	8	9	10	11	12	13
14	15	16	17	18	19	20
21	22	23	24	25	26	27
28	㉙	30				

Diana has been marking the first day of her period in her diary for 6 months. The first day of the period is day 1 of the menstrual cycle; therefore her cycle in April lasted 28 days, which is the average length. Since a month contains 30 or 31 days (except February), it is easy to see that sometimes a period will occur twice in a calendar month.

May

Sun	Mon	Tue	Wed	Thu	Fri	Sat
		1	2	3	4	
5	6	7	8	9	10	11
12	13	14	15	16	17	18
19	20	21	22	23	24	25
26	27	㉘	29	30	31	

Her next menstrual cycle started on April 29 and lasted for 29 days, until her period came again on May 28. Her subsequent cycles lasted 26, 28, 28, and 28 days, respectively. In summary, Diana's cycles vary from 26 to 28 days and are considered regular.

June

Sun	Mon	Tue	Wed	Thu	Fri	Sat
						1
2	3	4	5	6	7	8
9	10	11	12	13	14	15
16	17	18	19	20	21	22
㉓	24	25	26	27	28	29
30						

Her GP arranged for her progesterone level to be measured on the May 20, which was day 22 of her cycle. The result was 31 mmol/l which confirmed that she did ovulate.

July

Sun	Mon	Tue	Wed	Thu	Fri	Sat
	1	2	3	4	5	6
7	8	9	10	11	12	13
14	15	16	17	18	19	20
㉑	22	23	24	25	26	27
28	29	30	31			

August

Sun	Mon	Tue	Wed	Thu	Fri	Sat
				1	2	3
4	5	6	7	8	9	10
11	12	13	14	15	16	17
⑱	19	20	21	22	23	24
25	26	27	28	29	30	31

September

Sun	Mon	Tue	Wed	Thu	Fri	Sat
1	2	3	4	5	6	7
8	9	10	11	12	13	14
⑮	16	17	18	19	20	21
22	23	24	25	26	27	28
29	30					

Box 12.2 An irregular cycle

April

Sun	Mon	Tue	Wed	Thu	Fri	Sat
	①	2	3	4	5	6
7	8	9	10	11	12	13
14	15	16	17	18	19	20
21	22	23	24	25	26	27
28	29	30				

Susan has also been recording the first day of her period in order to calculate the length of her menstrual cycles. Although she had a period each calendar month except July, it can be seen that her cycle length is irregular, varying from 37 to 48 days (individual cycle lengths 40, 48, 37, and 44 days, respectively).

May

Sun	Mon	Tue	Wed	Thu	Fri	Sat
			1	2	3	4
5	6	7	8	9	10	⑪
12	13	14	15	16	17	18
19	20	21	22	23	24	25
26	27	28	29	30	31	

June

Sun	Mon	Tue	Wed	Thu	Fri	Sat
						1
2	3	4	5	6	7	8
9	10	11	12	13	14	15
16	17	18	19	20	21	22
23	24	25	26	27	㉘	29
30						

Susan had her progesterone measured on June 7 (day 28), June 14 (day 35), and June 21 (day 42); the measurements were 2 mmol/l, 4 mmol/l, and 3 mmol/l, respectively, indicating that she did not ovulate (i.e. she was having anovulatory cycles).

July

Sun	Mon	Tue	Wed	Thu	Fri	Sat
	1	2	3	4	5	6
7	8	9	10	11	12	13
14	15	16	17	18	19	20
21	22	23	24	25	26	27
28	29	30	31			

August

Sun	Mon	Tue	Wed	Thu	Fri	Sat
				1	2	3
④	5	6	7	8	9	10
11	12	13	14	15	16	17
18	19	20	21	22	23	24
25	26	27	28	29	30	31

September

Sun	Mon	Tue	Wed	Thu	Fri	Sat
1	2	3	4	5	6	7
8	9	10	11	12	13	14
15	16	⑰	18	19	20	21
22	23	24	25	26	27	28
29	30					

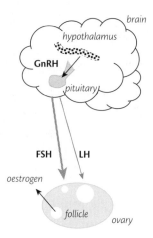

Figure 12.1 The control of ovulation. At the bigining of a normal menstrual cycle, a small group of follicles begin to grow in each ovary under the influence of the hormone FSH. FSH is released from the pituitary gland in the brain in response to another hormone called GnRH which is made by the hypothalamus. Eventually, one of these follicles becomes larger that the rest and is called the dominant follicle. A suddene surge of the hormone LH form the pituitary causes rapture of the follicle with the release of the mature egg (ovulation). Thus the two ovaries only release a egg between them each cycle

The control of ovulation

Ovulation is under the control of two hormones produced by the brain, follicle stimulating hormone (FSH) and luteinizing hormone (LH), as discussed in Chapter 3 and summarized in Figure 12.1. FSH and LH are carried in the bloodstream to the ovaries where they stimulate the growth of a follicle, which is the structure containing the egg, and trigger its release, which is called ovulation.

The developing follicle in the ovary produces a hormone called oestrogen. As the oestrogen level rises, it reduces the production of FSH by the pituitary. This is called a negative feedback mechanism and helps to control the amount of FSH released.

Causes of anovulation

Normal follicle development needs coordination of production of hormones from the brain and the ovary. The most common cause of anovulation is polycystic ovary syndrome, which is primarily an abnormality of the ovary.

Polycystic ovary syndrome (PCOS)

Symptoms of PCOS

PCOS is the most common hormone disorder in women of reproductive age, affecting approximately 7 per cent of women. Periods are usually irregular

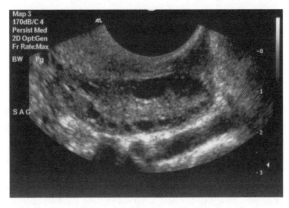

Figure 12.2 Ultrasound scan of a polycystic ovary. The polycystic ovary contains many more follicles than a normal ovary: these are visible as black "holes" on the ultrasound image. As in the normal ovary, each of these follicles potentially contains a microscopic egg which is too small to be seen. The polycystic ovary is usually larger than a normal ovary as well.

(indicating infrequent ovulation) and the ovaries contain an increased number of follicles, which can be seen on an ultrasound scan of the pelvis (Figure 12.2). It is the lack of regular ovulation in PCOS which causes infertility.

> ✖ **Myth:** Having polycystic ovaries means that your ovaries are full of cysts and you need an operation to remove them.
>
> ❗ **Fact:** These are not cysts but egg sacs.

The polycystic ovary also produces a slightly increased level of androgens (male hormones). These androgens (testosterone or androstenedione) can be measured with a blood test. Androgens can cause an increase in coarse, often dark, hair on the upper lip, chin, cheeks, and/or neck. It commonly causes a streak of hair below the umbilicus (tummy button) towards the pubic hair, which itself may extend sideways onto the thighs. Arm and leg hair may grow more densely and scattered hairs may grow around the nipples or be found on the chest and/or back. This pattern of excess hair growth is called hirsutism. The skin of the face, chest, and back may be excessively greasy, and stubborn acne affecting these areas is common. The extent of the hair growth and the severity of the acne varies. Another symptom caused by the increased androgens found in PCOS is frontal scalp hair loss.

The pattern of symptoms described above is often called the 'classic' picture of PCOS. Experts now recognize that there are some women with regular periods who ovulate regularly, but have acne or unwanted hair growth, and have poly-cystic ovaries. This is also called PCOS, but fertility in these women is likely to be normal.

Polycystic ovaries without symptoms

Some women have polycystic ovaries, but regular periods with normal ovula-tion and no symptoms associated with raised androgen levels. These women do NOT have polycystic ovary *syndrome*. Indeed, more than one in five normal women will have polycystic ovaries on ultrasound scan. However, the appear-ance of the ovary is important if fertility treatment to stimulate the ovaries is required. The large number of follicles present in polycystic ovaries, regardless of whether in association with the syndrome or not, means that the risk of ovarian hyperstimulation syndrome (OHSS) (see Chapter 15) occurring is higher than normal. In these circumstances, the dose of stimulating drugs used is usually adjusted to reduce the risk.

Anovulation in polycystic ovaries

It is not completely understood why some women with PCOS do not ovulate. These women tend to have slightly increased insulin levels compared with normal. High insulin levels can stop follicles from growing and as a result an egg is not released. Raised levels of the hormone LH, a common finding in PCOS, have a similar effect. Being overweight also raises insulin levels. When obesity and PCOS coexist, as they often do, the effects on insulin are additive; insulin levels are raised further and the frequency of ovulation is reduced even more. Typically, the effect of raised LH is more important in slim women with PCOS, whereas the effect of raised insulin is more significant in the overweight.

Hypothalamic–pituitary failure

As already discussed, ovulation is controlled by two parts of the brain, the hypothalamus and the pituitary (Figure 12.1). The hypothalamus is located centrally in the brain and controls the body's response to internal and external influences—for example, emotional or physical stress and starvation. The pituitary gland lies just below and in front of the hypothalamus, at a point mid-way between the eyes. The hypothalamus produces gonadotrophin-releasing hormone (GnRH) which instructs the pituitary to release FSH and LH.

At times of emotional or physical stress, the hypothalamus stops sending the correct GnRH signal to the pituitary gland. As a result, FSH and LH levels are too low to stimulate follicle growth and ovulation. This is called 'hypothalamic amenorrhoea', and common causes are excessive weight loss and high levels of exercise.

FSH and LH levels can also be too low if the pituitary gland itself is not functioning properly despite normal signals from the hypothalamus. The causes of this type of problem are all rare.

Premature ovarian failure

Premature ovarian failure, often referred to as premature menopause, is the result of a severe reduction in egg number ('reduced ovarian reserve'). This results in high levels of FSH and LH which are trying to 'drive' follicle development. Unfortunately, once the ovarian reserve is significantly reduced, normal follicle development does not occur and an egg may only be released occasionally or not at all. Sadly, there is no treatment which can restore ovulation or, indeed, the number of eggs within the ovary. However, pregnancy may be achieved by fertilizing eggs that have been collected from a donor (see Chapter 18).

Other hormone problems

Low levels of the hormone thyroxin, produced by the thyroid gland found at the base of the neck, can cause failure of ovulation. Ovarian function can be restored by correcting the imbalance with thyroid supplements (thyroxine). Thyroxine is important for the normal development of the baby during pregnancy and your doctor will check your thyroid levels regularly as it is often necessary to increase your level of thyroxine when you are pregnant.

High levels of the hormone prolactin, which is also produced by the pituitary gland and is best known for stimulating the production of milk in the breast, can also interfere with ovulation. Prolactin levels can be lowered with bromocriptine or cabergoline; both drugs are safe to take whilst trying to get pregnant. Since it is normal for prolactin levels to rise during pregnancy (and indeed necessary to prepare the breast for producing milk after delivery), your doctor will advise you when to stop taking bromocriptine/cabergoline once pregnancy has been confirmed.

Table 12.1 Hormone levels associated with the most common causes of anovulation

Diagnosis	FSH levels	LH levels	Oestrogen levels
PCOS	Normal	High	Normal
Hypothalamic amenorrhoea	Low	Low	Low
Premature ovarian failure	High	Normal or high	Low
High prolactin	Low	Low	Low

Ovaries normally produce the hormone oestrogen and the amount of oestrogen produced is related to the number of follicles growing in the ovary. In PCOS, there are a large number of small follicles and oestrogen levels are therefore normal. In premature ovarian failure, hypothalamic amenorrhoea and high prolactin, there are very few growing follicles of any size and oestrogen levels are low.

13

Ovulation induction

 Key points

- Treatment of ovulation problems is highly successful in PCOS.

- Overweight women with PCOS can increase their frequency of ovulation by moderate weight loss. Women with a body mass index (BMI) greater than 30 are unlikely to respond to drugs used to induce ovulation.

- Clomifene is usually the first drug of choice.

- Approximately 10 per cent of pregnancies conceived via clomifene administration will be multiple pregnancies.

- Alternatives to clomifene treatment for women with PCOS are FSH injections and laparoscopic ovarian drilling.

Ovulation induction (OI), as the term suggests, is treatment for anovulation. Strictly speaking, OI is not actually a form of assisted reproduction as it is simply aiming to mimic the normal activity of the ovary, thereby allowing spontaneous pregnancy. There are various different treatment options for inducing ovulation, depending on the underlying problem. However, the aim of ovulation induction is always the same—to allow the release of one egg per treatment cycle.

Weight loss

Women with PCOS who are overweight can increase their frequency of ovulation by losing weight. The effect of being overweight on the polycystic ovary was discussed in the previous chapter. Importantly, even moderate weight loss (5–10 per cent of starting weight) results in more frequent episodes of ovulation. Women with a body mass index (BMI) of over 30 (calculated as weight in kilograms divided by height in metres squared) are also unlikely to respond to the drugs used to induce ovulation. Weight loss will improve the response to these methods as well as lowering the health risks to both mother and baby in pregnancy.

Weight gain

Being underweight can be as harmful to fertility as being overweight (see Chapter 12). Weight gain will eventually allow the brain to send the correct signals to the pituitary gland which in turn communicates with the ovaries (see Chapter 12, Figure 12.1). However, there may be a considerable time lag between weight gain and the return of ovulation (months to a couple of years) and it is important to maintain weight during this time. Similarly, if excessive amounts of exercise are being undertaken, particularly aerobic activities such as running, reduction will improve ovarian activity.

Clomifene (Clomid)

Clomifene works by indirectly stimulating the growth of one or more follicles within the ovaries. It is an excellent treatment for women with PCOS who do not release eggs, and is usually the drug of first choice for these women if their BMI is under 30. Ovulation will occur in 90 per cent. Clomifene is a tablet which is taken once a day for 5 days, usually beginning between days 2 and 5 of the period. If periods are very infrequent, progesterone tablets will usually be given first to induce one.

It is very important that the response of the ovaries to clomifene is monitored until the correct dose is achieved. An ultrasound scan is normally performed before ovulation is anticipated, usually around days 10–12 of the cycle. This is to ensure that one (or at most two) follicles are growing. The thickness of the endometrium (womb lining) is also measured at this time. If there is no obvious dominant follicle, the scan will be repeated, usually twice a week, until around day 22. At that point, if there is still no follicle developing, progesterone tablets will be given to induce a period and the clomifene treatment will be repeated at a higher dose. The usual maximum dose of clomifene is two tablets (100 mg) a day for 5 days, although some specialists may recommend up to three tablets (150 mg) at a time.

If one or two follicles are seen to be growing, ovulation will be confirmed with a blood test to measure progesterone levels approximately a week after it was estimated to occur. Once this has been confirmed, the same dose of clomifene can be repeated for six to nine cycles.

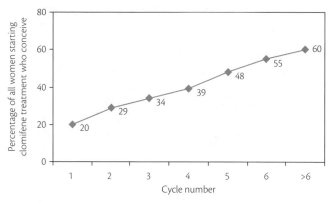

Figure 13.1 Cumulative pregnancy rates with clomifene. The first point on the graph shows the number of couples who conceived after the one cycle of treatment. The second point shows the number who conceived after the first cycle plus the second cycle and so on. Only a small number of couples conceive after 6 cycles of treatment. Data from E Kousta, D White & S Franks, Imperial College London

What if too many follicles grow?

If three or more follicles in total are growing on the ovaries, the cycle should be abandoned with either abstinence from sex or the use of a condom for the following week. This is because of an increased risk of a multiple pregnancy—twins, triplets, or more! Approximately 10 per cent of pregnancies conceived on clomifene will be multiple pregnancies which, sadly, are associated with increased risks to to both mother and babies.

What if clomiphene treatment doesn't work?

Although 90 per cent of women with PCOS will ovulate on clomifene, after up to nine cycles of treatment only 60 per cent of them will be pregnant (20 per cent conceive on the first cycle). Very few pregnancies occur in women who take more than nine cycles of clomifene, which is why treatment is usually discontinued at that point.

> If 100 women with PCOS start ovulation induction, 90 will ovulate and 54 will be pregnant after up to nine cycles of treatment.

Occasionally, clomifene can prevent the endometrium (womb lining) from thickening normally even though ovulation is occurring. You may be recommended

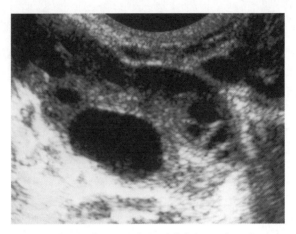

Figure 13.2 Ultrasound scan of a pre-ovulatory follicle in a polycystic ovary

another method of ovulation induction if this happens. Sometimes a drug called tamoxifen is recommended. It is actually related to clomifene; in fact the two molecules are mirror-images of each other and they work in the same way. However, in some women tamoxifen may allow the endometrium to thicken when this has not happened with clomifene.

There are two alternative treatments to clomifene (and tamoxifen) which can be used with good effect if clomifene has failed to induce ovulation (clomifene resistance) or if ovulatory cycles, with normal development of the womb lining, have been established but pregnancy has not occurred.

FSH injections

One option is daily injections with the hormone FSH. Because of the impact of obesity on ovarian function, most units will insist that the BMI is under 28 before starting this treatment. Different clinics use different preparations (some contain only FSH and others also contain small amounts of LH) but all have to be injected once a day. There is no proven benefit of any particular preparation. Apart from the inconvenience of daily injections, the main drawback of this treatment is that ultrasound scans of the ovaries are required once or twice a week throughout treatment. This is because of the potentially serious complication of ovarian hyperstimulation syndrome (OHSS) (see Chapter 15) which is very rare with clomifene.

The starting dose of FSH is very low, and during the first cycle of treatment it is increased at fortnightly intervals until one or two dominant follicles are seen to be growing on ultrasound scan. Once the follicle(s) is large enough to

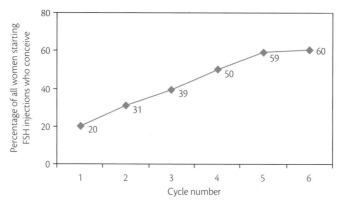

Figures 13.3 Cumulative pregnancy rates with FSH injections in women who are either clomiphene resistant or who did not conceive after 9 cycles of clomifene. 60% of women treated with FSH injections will conceive over up to 6 cycles, again 20% of pregnancies will be in the 1st cycle of treatment. Pregnancies are rare with this treatment in women who have not conceived after 6 cycles. Data from A Gorry, D White & S Franks, Imperial College Healthcare NHS Trust

release the egg (usually when 16–18 mm in diameter), a different injection, of a hormone called human chorionic gonadotrophin (hCG), is given and this triggers ovulation approximately 36 hours later.

For the same reasons as during clomifene treatment, the cycle is abandoned if three or more follicles are growing. Approximately 10 per cent of cycles have to be cancelled because of this.

> Of 100 women starting treatment, there will be 46 women who did not conceive after clomifene (either because of clomifene resistance or no pregnancy despite ovulation), 27 will conceive over six cycles with FSH injections.

Laparoscopic ovarian drilling

Laparoscopic ovarian drilling (LOD) is an operation to increase the chance of ovulation. It can be offered as an alternative to FSH injections or after six ovulatory cycles if pregnancy has not occurred. The aim of LOD is to promote spontaneous ovulation, or to convert a woman who is clomifene resistant into one who is clomiphene sensitive. Ideally, a woman's BMI should be under 30 for this treatment. Sometimes LOD is recommended before trying clomifene treatment, for example if the doctor feels that it is important to examine your pelvis laparoscopically (see Chapter 7) or if there are strong reasons to avoid the risk of multiple pregnancy.

LOD involves an operation called a laparoscopy which is done under general anaesthetic (see Chapter 7 for a more detailed discussion of laparoscopy and its risks). During the laparoscopy, between four and ten 'holes' are burnt into the surface of each ovary using a fine needle heated with an electric current (diathermy). An alternative method is to use a laser beam at laparoscopy; the effects are the same. It is not really understood how this method promotes ovulation, but it is probably due to transient alterations in hormone levels caused by the destruction of ovarian tissue.

After LOD, cycle monitoring should be performed to confirm if ovulation has been successfully induced or not. If ovulation is not occurring, clomifene treatment can be attempted again. Pregnancy rates are approximately the same 6–12 months after LOD as after up to six cycles of FSH injections.

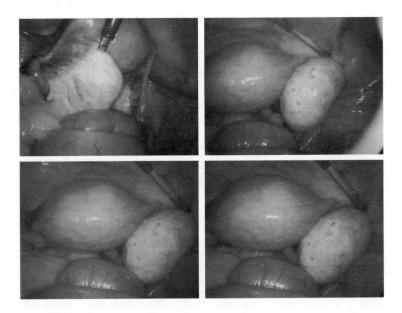

Figure 13.4 Laparoscopic ovarian diathermy. Using keyhole surgery, the ovary is 'drilled' with an electrically-heated needle. The number of holes made varies with the size of the ovary, but four in each ovary is average.

Table 13.1 Advantages and disadvantages of ovulation induction methods for PCOS

Treatment	Advantage	Disadvantage
Clomifene	90% ovulation rate 60% pregnancy rate Very low risk of OHSS Convenient treatment	10% multiple pregnancy rate Womb lining (endometrium) may be made thin Cervical mucus may be less welcoming to sperm
FSH injections	60% pregnancy rate	7.5% multiple pregnancy rate Moderate risk of OHSS Frequent scans and blood tests Daily injections 18% of cycles cancelled
LOD	The effect of one treatment episode may last several years No monitoring required once ovulation demonstrated No increased risk of multiple pregnancy May now respond to clomiphene Pelvis can be assessed fully at time of procedure Pregnancy rates approximately the same as for FSH injections	Risks of surgery Risks of general anaesthetic Clomiphene or FSH injections may still be required after LOD
Metformin	No increased risk of multiple pregnancy No monitoring required once ovulation demonstrated	Low rate of ovulation Low rate of pregnancy per ovulation Limited safety data for use in early pregnancy Stomach upsets

Metformin

Metformin is a drug that is used to treat diabetes. It works by making the body more sensitive to insulin, thereby lowering insulin levels. Because of this effect on insulin, metformin can promote ovulation in women with PCOS. However, ovulation rates are very low in comparison to clomifene, and the chance of pregnancy per ovulation is much lower with metformin treatment than with clomiphene. In addition, many women are unable to tolerate the drug, as it often causes nausea, diarrhoea, abdominal cramps, and bloating. Its main attraction is that there is no increased risk of multiple pregnancy, reducing the need for monitoring. Whilst metformin may have a role for a small number of women with PCOS, most specialists in PCOS now feel that it is not a particularly useful treatment.

Metformin is also sometimes prescribed to help women with PCOS to lose weight. In fact, there is no good evidence that it actually works for this purpose. Some women do lose weight whilst taking metformin, but that is probably because they are eating less as a result of the stomach upsets that it causes.

GnRH pump

When anovulation is due to abnormal production of GnRH by the hypothalamus (see Chapter 12, Figure 12.1), replacing GnRH drives the release of FSH and LH from the pituitary. This in turn stimulates follicle growth and so ovulation. The major advantage of this treatment is that when ovulation does occur, it almost invariably results in the release of only one egg per cycle and multiple pregnancy rates are no higher than in the general population (less than 2 per cent). However, it is less successful at inducing ovulation in PCOS. The major drawback of this treatment is that the drug has to be given by a pump which automatically delivers a small dose every 60–90 minutes via a needle placed just below the skin. The needle can stay in place for several days and the pump, which is about the size of an MP3 player/iPOD, is strapped to the arm and worn continuously.

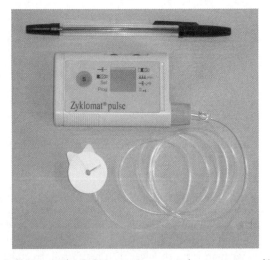

Figure 13.5 GnRH pump. The GnRH pump is worn on the upper arm and is battery operated. The tubing connects the vial of hormone to a fine needle which is inserted through the skin of the arm and is held in place by the white dressing. The pump releases a small amount of drug every 60 to 90 minutes, depending on the setting selected by the doctor. (The pen is there for scale). Reproduced with permission of Ferring Pharmaceuticals.

For some women, despite the inconvenience of wearing the pump, the advantage of a low risk of multiple pregnancy make this an attractive treatment option. For others, FSH injections, which "by-pass" the requirement for GnRH, are preferable.

Table 13.2 Methods of ovulation induction for common causes of anovulation

Diagnosis	Clomiphene	FSH	GnRH pump	LOD
PCOS	√	√	X	√
Hypothalamic amenorrhoea	×	√	√	×
Premature ovarian failure	×	×	×	×

> Clomifene is the first-line treatment for PCOS as it is convenient, successful and is low risk. Laparoscopic ovarian drilling is only ever used for PCOS. Sadly, when anovulation is due to reduced ovarian reserve/premature ovarian failure, none of these treatments will work.

The role of IVF in anovulatory disorders

IVF is rarely required by women who do not ovulate because of the success of ovulation induction treatments (the exception being anovulation caused by severely reduced ovarian reserve/premature ovarian failure). However, after six to nine cycles of clomiphene treatment followed by 6 months of FSH injections, or 6–12 months after LOD, most couples are advised to move on to IVF. The comparatively low pregnancy rates per cycle of superovulation with intrauterine insemination make this option unrealistic for most couples who may have already had up to 2 years of ovulation induction treatment.

Summary

Anovulation explains approximately 20 per cent of infertility. The most common cause of anovulation is PCOS. Unless the cause is reduced ovarian reserve/premature ovarian failure, ovulation induction has a high chance of success. It is usual to look for other causes of infertility (e.g. to check that the tubes are open and the sperm count is normal) even when anovulation has been identified.

14

In vitro fertilization (including ICSI and IVM)

> ## Key points
>
> ◆ *In vitro* fertilization (IVF) involves joining the egg and sperm outside the body. It is often described as 'test-tube baby' treatment.
>
> ◆ The first test-tube baby, Louise Brown, was born in the UK in 1978.
>
> ◆ IVF is recommended for women with damaged Fallopian tubes or for men with very low sperm counts or poorly moving sperm. It is also indicated for couples with unexplained infertility if they have been trying for a long time.
>
> ◆ Although NHS funding may be available, most IVF treatment in the UK is self-funded.
>
> ◆ In the UK, about one in four treatment cycles of IVF leads to a successful birth.

What is IVF?

IVF stands for *in vitro* fertilization—joining the egg and sperm outside the body. It is often called 'test-tube baby' treatment.

The first test-tube baby, Louise Brown, was born in Britain in 1978. This followed years of preparatory work by gynaecologist Patrick Steptoe and scientist Robert Edwards, who pioneered IVF despite opposition from the medical and scientific establishment and criticism that it was unethical to 'create' human life. However, over the last 30 years, IVF has become so successful and such a common form of treatment that at least one in 100 pregnancies in the UK are conceived this way. About 10 000 IVF babies have been born in the UK.

Will I need IVF?

Before deciding to have IVF, infertile couples should have investigations and discuss their options with a doctor who is experienced in treating infertility.

Depending on the cause of infertility, there may be simpler treatments that would be effective. These are discussed in separate chapters.

IVF is the best form of treatment for women with damaged Fallopian tubes, where a blockage prevents the eggs and sperm from meeting. Surgical repair of the tubes is less successful (except for very minor damage, or reversal of sterilization). IVF is also recommended if scarring or 'adhesions' around the tubes and ovaries prevents the eggs from getting down the tubes, for example after a burst appendix or severe endometriosis.

Men with very low sperm counts or poorly moving sperm will also best be treated with IVF. They may need a special technique called ICSI (see below).

IVF is also recommended for couples with unexplained infertility if they have been trying for a long time (certainly if they have been trying for over 5 years) or the woman is older than 35. Couples may also need to move on to IVF when simpler treatments have been tried without success.

Is it easy to obtain treatment? Will I have to pay?

In the UK there are currently over 70 fertility clinics that offer IVF, so there is likely to be a clinic within reach of you. A full list of licensed units, addresses, and contact details can be obtained from the HFEA (see Useful addresses).

NHS funding may be available for treatment. In 2004 the government declared support for the provision of IVF through the NHS, with the aim of funding up to three cycles of IVF for couples needing it. However, this is only available in a few areas, and the level of funding still varies widely across the UK depending on your local primary care trust or health board. Most areas fund some IVF, but there can be long waiting lists for treatment. There will also be restrictions, for example on age—NHS funds are not given to women after their 40th birthday. Treatment is usually only available to couples without children. You will be treated at your local hospital or at a local private clinic under a special arrangement with the NHS.

Most IVF treatment in the UK is self-funded. Costs vary widely and tend to be higher in London and in units that are entirely private. A single cycle of IVF can cost from £3000 to £8000. Usually the clinic will charge an all-inclusive fee to cover all the medical treatment, but you need to check whether there will be additional costs; for example, you may need preliminary tests. The drugs will need to be purchased on prescription and can be very expensive. The HFEA levies a fee of about £100 per cycle of IVF to cover the costs of inspecting and licensing clinics, and many clinics pass this on to the patient.

Private treatment is usually available without delay. You can choose which clinic you want to attend (see Chapter 4 for advice on choosing a clinic).

Myth: IVF takes months and months.

 Fact: IVF requires some initial investigations and preparation, but the actual time between starting fertility injections and egg collection is about 2 weeks.

What does the treatment involve?

Preparation

Before starting treatment you will need a consultation to discuss IVF. Both partners should attend this. Some units (particularly in the NHS) run group sessions to explain the procedures. You will both be asked to complete forms giving your consent to disclose information about your treatment, for example to your GP, and a 'Welfare of the Child' form giving information on your social circumstances which might have a bearing on your ability to bring up a child.

The IVF unit will need all the information on your previous tests and treatment. If you are having treatment in the private sector it may be your responsibility to provide these; you can request copies of your test results from your GP or hospital clinic. This will avoid repeating tests unnecessarily.

Men will be asked to give a semen sample for analysis before treatment starts, often at the first visit. Women will need to have an ultrasound scan to check that the ovaries are accessible for egg collection. Most units will also update the tests of ovarian function; this may involve a blood test and scan on day 3 of the cycle before starting any medication. This helps to calculate the dose of drugs that will be needed. Some units will also check the inside of the womb and carry out a 'dummy' embryo transfer to make sure that that there will be no problems on the day of treatment.

Medication

Several types of medication are used in IVF treatment and you will be given a schedule of when and how to take them. The IVF unit will write the prescription for you, and they will usually have stocks of medication so that you can obtain it from them. If you are paying for your treatment, you may wish to 'shop around' to see whether you can buy it more cheaply. It is unlikely that your GP will be able to help you obtain the prescription through the NHS.

Your clinic may ask you to take one packet of contraceptive pill or a course of progesterone tablets during the month before your IVF treatment to control the ovaries and make sure that your period starts on time.

Injections are used to stimulate the ovaries to produce plenty of eggs. These contain gonadotrophins or FSH (follicle-stimulating hormone), which are hormones made naturally during the monthly cycle. The injections are usually started during the period and given for 10–12 days. They are given once a day, at roughly the same time. The injections go just under the skin, and most couples are able to do this at home (if you know anyone with diabetes who needs to take insulin, the injections are very similar). Several brands are available from different drug companies, but they are all equally effective.

A second medicine is given to prevent your body reacting too quickly to the treatment and ovulating early. If you were to ovulate before the egg collection, all the eggs would be 'lost'. There are two ways of doing this: a drug called GnRH analogue is given as a nasal spray or injection which may be started before your period or during the period; alternatively, an injection of GnRH antagonist is given alongside the stimulating injection. Both these drugs block the release of the hormone that triggers ovulation.

You may hear the terms 'short protocol', 'flare protocol', 'long protocol', or 'mid-luteal protocol'. These terms all refer to the timing of the medication, and whether the blocking drug is given alongside the stimulating injections (short/ flare), before them (long), or in the previous cycle (mid-luteal).

When the follicles (egg sacs) have reached the correct size, a final injection is given which matures the eggs. This contains hCG, which mimics the hormone LH that causes ovulation. The clinic will give you instructions on the timing of this injection, which is usually given in the evening 36 hours before the eggs are collected.

Following embryo transfer, hormone supplements are given to build up the womb lining and improve the chance of a pregnancy implanting. You may be prescribed progesterone in the form of vaginal pessaries or injections.

Antibiotics may be given around the time of egg collection to reduce the small risk of infection from the procedure. Men may also be asked to take antibiotics to reduce the chance of any infection in the semen sample.

Research is being carried out on some other medicines that might be helpful in implantation, including aspirin and blood-thinning injections. At present, we do not have proof that these are effective and so they cannot be recommended for routine use. There can be serious side effects from steroid tablets and immuno-globulin (IVIG) injections, and these should be avoided.

Monitoring

Your response to the medication will be watched closely. You will have vaginal ultrasound scans to count the number of eggs developing and measure the size of the follicles, and you may also have blood tests for oestrogen levels. Depending on the results, the dose of the injections may be changed accordingly, and the day of egg collection will be confirmed. Occasionally a cycle may be cancelled if there are not enough eggs to go ahead with collection.

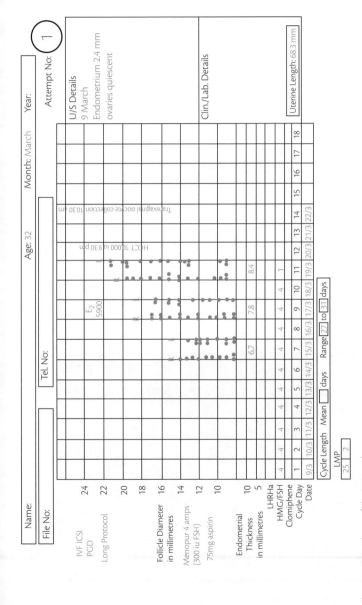

Figure 14.1 Chart of the IVF cycle.

Egg collection

The eggs are collected from the ovaries guided by vaginal ultrasound. The scan machine has a special probe with a needle, which is passed through the skin of the vagina. The ovaries are very close to the top of the vagina and can be seen on the screen. The tip of the needle is visible as it enters each follicle (egg sac) in turn, and the fluid inside is sucked out into a test-tube. This is checked under a microscope to find the eggs.

The egg collection takes about half-an-hour. It is done under sedation or light anaesthesia. You will be asked to come to the clinic early in the morning, having had nothing to eat or drink beforehand. You will probably be able to leave in the early afternoon.

Eggs can also be collected using laparoscopy with a telescope inserted in the abdomen under general anaesthesia. This is uncommon nowadays.

A semen sample, which is is used to fertilize the eggs, will be needed on the day of egg collection.

Embryo transfer

You will be asked to return to the clinic 2–6 days after egg collection. The laboratory will let you know how many eggs have fertilized and developed, and they may be able to show you the embryos on a screen. Having the embryo transfer is an outpatient procedure and it is rare to need anaesthesia. You may be asked to have a full bladder, and an ultrasound scan may be done. The doctor will place an

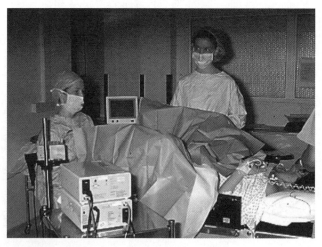

Figure 14.2 Egg collection procedure.

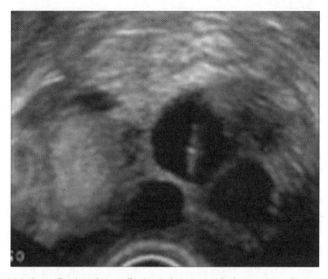

Figure 14.3 Egg collection: the needle tip can be seen inside the ovary on ultrasound scan.

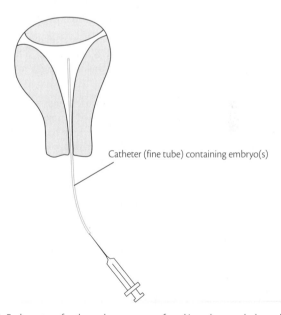

Catheter (fine tube) containing embryo(s)

Figure 14.4 Embryo transfer: the embryos are transferred into the womb through the cervix.

instrument in the vagina (like having a smear test), and then clean the cervix and gently pass a fine tube through the opening into the womb. The embryo(s) are placed high in the womb. You may be asked to rest in the clinic for 30 minutes before leaving.

Are there any risks?

The main risk to women going through IVF treatment is overstimulation by the injections. This is called 'ovarian hyperstimulation syndrome' (OHSS) and is described in Chapter 15.

The risk of OHSS is highest in women with polycystic ovaries and women who become pregnant. If OHSS is starting to develop, the drug dosage can be adjusted; in a few cases it may be necessary to avoid embryo transfer and freeze all embryos. OHSS cannot always be prevented. One or two in a hundred women having IVF will need to be admitted to hospital for treatment of OHSS.

Multiple pregnancy (carrying two or more babies) carries risks to both the mother and the children, as explained in Chapter 24. The mother is more likely to suffer from complications in pregnancy, such as high blood pressure and diabetes, and to be delivered by Caesarean operation. Twins and triplets are almost always born prematurely, and they are smaller at birth than a singleton baby. As a result, they are far more likely to die or suffer disability.

The risks of multiple pregnancy can be avoided by replacing only a single embryo at a time in IVF treatment. Current UK regulations allow transfer of just two embryos, and there are plans to limit this to a single embryo in some circumstances.

There has been concern that stimulation of the ovaries might be a risk factor for ovarian cancer, and that the high hormone levels of oestrogen might increase the risk of breast cancer. However, thousands of women have been followed up without showing any definite increase in cancer due to fertility treatment. Women who do not have children have a higher lifetime chance of ovarian cancer.

What is the success rate of IVF?

In the UK about one in four treatment cycles leads to a successful birth. The success rate depends on the woman's age: the chance of live birth is 28 per cent for women under 35, but falls to 11 per cent for women aged 40–42 and drops below 5 per cent for women over 42. Currently, about one in four IVF births in the UK are twins. This figure should fall over the next few years as single-embryo transfer becomes more common.

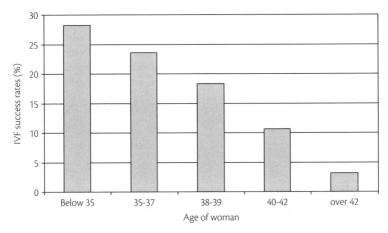

Figure 14.5 IVF success (percentage live births per cycle started) according to the woman's age (drawn from HFEA data on UK treatment cycles 2003–2004).

Success rates in the UK are published every year by the HFEA (www.hfea.gov. uk). Every clinic must report every IVF cycle to the HFEA—currently about 40 000 each year—showing how many cycles led to embryo transfer, how many pregnancies were achieved, and how many births (of course the birth figures come a year later).

Individual clinics can publish their own rates in more detail. Comparing clinics is not always useful; success rates will be affected by the type of patients they treat. One clinic might look 'better' than another, but because the actual number of treatments in each clinic is small there may be no real statistical difference between them.

Can IVF treatment be repeated?

Yes: if your first IVF cycle does not succeed, talk to your clinic and get advice about further treatment. There is an element of luck, and for most couples it is worth trying again. Rather like throwing dice, if you do it repeatedly you will eventually throw a six. However, sometimes it becomes clear during treatment that IVF is not likely to succeed—for example, if very few eggs of poor quality are collected. You need to be given realistic advice.

You will need to have a break of at least a month between IVF treatment cycles, and preferably longer, to allow the ovaries to settle down. Otherwise the response to stimulation in the next cycle will not be as good.

NHS funding for repeated cycles is very limited in most areas.

What happens in the laboratory?

When the eggs are collected, they are put into a labelled dish and incubated in fluid at body temperature to finish maturing. The semen sample taken on the same day is analysed and prepared so that the moving sperm are extracted. A droplet containing many thousands of sperm is added to each egg.

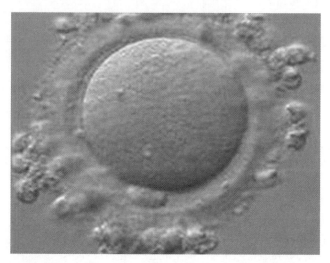

Figure 14.6 Human egg.

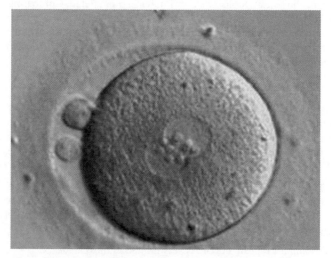

Figure 14.7 Fertilized egg (also called a 'zygote'). The genetic material is visible in the centre.

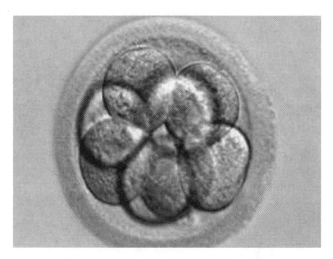

Figure 14.8 Eight-cell embryo.

The following day, the eggs are examined under the microscope for signs of fertilization, when a sperm penetrates the egg (Figure 14.7). Not all eggs are likely to be healthy, but usually two-thirds of them will fertilize. When this occurs, the genetic material from the man and the woman fuses and the cell starts to divide. The dividing bundle of cells is called an embryo.

The embryos are examined to check their progress. Not all of them will survive and grow to the stage where they can be replaced into the womb. The embryology staff will 'grade' the embryos and select the best to replace (Figure 14.8).

Special techniques in IVF

ICSI (intra-cytoplasmic sperm injection) is a specialist laboratory technique. A single sperm is picked up under the microscope and injected into the centre of an egg (Figure 14.9). This fertilizes the egg even if the sperm is too weak to penetrate it naturally. This technique was developed in the 1990s, after an accidental discovery, and it transformed the outlook for men with low sperm counts who otherwise could not father a child. Currently, ICSI is undertaken in more than four in ten cycles of IVF in the UK.

Assisted hatching is a laboratory technique which may improve the chances of an embryo implanting into the womb, but it is not yet proven to be of value. The human egg is surrounded by an outer coat called the 'zona pellucida', in the same way that a hen's egg is surrounded by a shell. After a sperm has penetrated and fertilized the egg, the embryo grows and divides until it breaks out through the zona and burrows into the wall of the womb. In assisted hatching a hole is created in the zona to make it easier for the embryo to emerge.

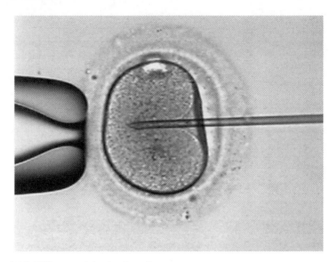

Figure 14.9 ICSI: sperm injection into the egg.

Blastocyst transfer is increasingly used if couples have several embryos to choose from. The embryos are kept for longer than usual in the laboratory—5 or 6 days rather than 2 or 3 days. The healthiest surviving embryos will reach the blastocyst stage. These are believed to have the best potential for pregnancy and are selected for transfer to the womb.

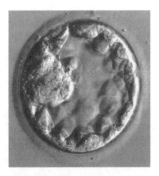

Figure 14.10 Blastocyst.

Embryo biopsy means the removal of one or two cells for analysis. These are usually taken from the developing embryo at the eight-cell stage. Embryo biopsy is done for preimplantation genetic diagnosis (see Chapter 16).

IVM (*in vitro* maturation) is a process whereby immature eggs are collected from the ovaries, matured in the laboratory, and then fertilized. This avoids the need for ovarian stimulation. It is most suitable for women with polycystic ovaries who are at high risk of OHSS. It will potentially be very useful for women suffering from cancer who wish to store eggs but do not have enough time for standard IVF. Currently, only a few hundred babies have been born worldwide, and IVM is only just being introduced in the UK. Further information is needed on long-term safety, but no risks have been identified.

GIFT

GIFT (gamete intra-Fallopian transfer) is an assisted conception treatment which can be an alternative to IVF. The ovaries are stimulated in the same way and the eggs are collected, but they are immediately replaced in the Fallopian tubes together with a prepared sperm sample. This is done by laparoscopy (keyhole surgery) under general anaesthetic. Fertilization then takes place inside the body.

GIFT used to be a popular treatment before the laboratory techniques of IVF were widely available. It is not commonly used now, but remains a possible treatment for unexplained infertility. Some clinics find that it gives better success rates than IVF for older women or those with poor egg quality, presumably because the eggs thrive better in their natural environment.

ZIFT (zygote intra-Fallopian transfer) is an IVF cycle with transfer of the embryos to the Fallopian tubes by laparoscopy. It is uncommon, but may be recommended if embryo transfer through the cervix is very difficult.

Natural cycle IVF

IVF can be carried out without stimulating drugs in a natural menstrual cycle. Although Louise Brown was born this way, it is not a very successful technique— it is difficult to extract, fertilize, and grow just one egg.

Of course, many couples are keen to avoid the use of drug treatment, and 'minimal stimulation' IVF is becoming popular. This means that mild fertility drugs are used which will result in three or four eggs. The treatment for the woman is simpler and does not carry much risk of OHSS. It can probably be repeated more frequently than conventional IVF. More evidence on the success rates of mild IVF is still needed.

Embryo freezing

Spare embryos can be frozen and stored to give a chance for couples to have a second child, or to try again if the first transfer does not succeed. Embryos are stored at a very low temperature in liquid nitrogen, so that they do not deteriorate over time. The storage period is usually 5 years, but this can be extended. Not all embryos will survive freezing and thawing, and the success rate of treatment is lower than with fresh embryos. However, it is still a valuable option as it avoids the need to repeat ovarian stimulation.

The first birth from frozen-thawed embryos was in 1984, and at least 250 000 babies have been estimated to have been born worldwide using this technique. Many are siblings from the same batch of embryos, born several years apart. There is reassuring data on the safety of the technique.

Embryo freezing can be used by women who are diagnosed with cancer to preserve their chance of having children. As long as there is enough time before chemotherapy or radiotherapy treatment commences, an IVF cycle is started and all the embryos are frozen for future use. This is only applicable to women who are in a committed relationship, because both partners are involved in IVF treatment and in the future both partners have to give their consent before the embryos can be used.

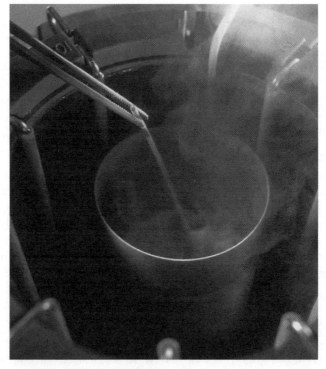

Figure 14.11 Frozen embryos in liquid nitrogen.

Frozen-thawed embryo transfer

The thawed embryos are placed into the womb on the correct day of the monthly cycle. This can be a natural cycle; you will be asked to do home urine tests for the LH surge and attend the clinic for one or two ultrasound scans to confirm the day of treatment. If the menstrual cycle is not regular or monitoring does not confirm a perfect cycle, hormone supplements will be used. This involves suppression of the natural cycle (usually with nasal spray) and tablets or patches of oestrogen for 2 weeks until the womb lining thickens, followed by progesterone pessaries or injections. The embryos are thawed and transferred on the equivalent day of the artificial cycle.

Egg freezing

Eggs can be frozen for storage without being fertilized. This still needs ovarian stimulation and egg collection, exactly as described above for an IVF cycle. Women without a male partner can freeze eggs for social reasons, as an insurance policy, or to preserve their fertility before cancer treatment.

Egg freezing is technically more difficult than embryo freezing and is less successful. Although research on frozen eggs has been extensive, the technique did not develop until the late 1990s and only a few hundred babies have been born around the world. There are exciting developments in the laboratory technique of egg freezing (vitrification) which may improve this.

15

Ovarian hyperstimulation

> ## ➔ Key points
>
> ◆ Ovarian hyperstimulation (OHSS) is a condition which only occurs in women receiving fertility drugs, usually gonadotrophins.
>
> ◆ OHSS is most likely to happen during IVF treatment cycles, usually after embryo transfer but sometimes earlier, around the time of egg collection.
>
> ◆ Women who have polycystic ovaries are more likely to develop OHSS. Younger women (aged less than 35 years) and slim women are more likely to be at risk of OHSS than those who are older or overweight.
>
> ◆ Women who suffer from severe OHSS are often pregnant. There is no evidence that OHSS causes any abnormalities in pregnancy, and the pregnancy should continue normally.
>
> ◆ It is important for those suspected of having OHSS to be seen by a specialist.

What is ovarian hyperstimulation?

Ovarian hyperstimulation syndrome (also called OHSS) is an illness that can occur in women receiving fertility drug treatment. The ovaries become enlarged and tender. Fluid can build up in the abdomen and sometimes around the lungs. This may require hospital admission and treatment until the symptoms settle down. The condition may last a few days or a few weeks. Although many women going through IVF have mild symptoms, severe OHSS is not common. About one or two in 100 women may need hospital admission. OHSS is more likely to occur in women who become pregnant.

What causes OHSS?

OHSS only occurs in women receiving fertility drugs, usually gonadotrophins. An excessive response to these drugs makes many small egg sacs (follicles) develop.

It is believed that the stimulated ovaries release chemical substances which make small blood vessels more porous. Fluid leaks out of these small blood vessels, leading to dehydration. The fluid accumulates in the abdominal cavity and, in more severe cases, around the lungs and even the heart. A serious but rare complication is thrombosis (blood clot), and the function of the kidneys, liver, and lungs can be affected. A small number of deaths (less than five in the UK) have been reported from complications of OHSS.

If pregnancy occurs following the fertility treatment, the hormone changes of early pregnancy can prolong the illness.

Am I at risk of OHSS?

Anyone receiving fertility drugs could be at risk of OHSS, and if you are having IVF treatment, you need to be aware of the symptoms. Your fertility unit should be able to give you information on OHSS.

OHSS is most likely to happen during IVF treatment cycles, usually after embryo transfer but sometimes earlier, around the time of egg collection. It can occur, but is rare, when injected fertility drugs (gonadotrophins) are given for superovulation or ovulation induction. It is very rare indeed with milder fertility drugs that are given as tablets (clomifene).

Women who have polycystic ovaries are more likely to develop OHSS. They may produce a large number of eggs in response to fertility drugs. Younger women (aged under 35) and slim women are more likely to be at risk of OHSS than those who are older or overweight.

What are the symptoms?

The first symptoms are swelling of the abdomen, pain in the lower abdomen, and nausea. Mild symptoms of abdominal bloating and tenderness are fairly common and occur in at least a third of women going through IVF, but you should seek advice if these become worse.

Contact the fertility unit if you feel breathless, if you have severe swelling or pain in the abdomen, if you are vomiting, or if you are passing less urine than usual and it looks dark or concentrated.

What should I do?

Symptoms of mild OHSS can be helped by resting and taking mild painkillers. Paracetamol is safe to take even though you might be pregnant. Avoid sexual intercourse and any strenuous exercise because the ovaries are very swollen and they might bleed. Try to drink enough clear fluids to avoid dehydration. Thirst is a good guide as to whether you are drinking enough.

OHSS usually develops after egg collection and embryo transfer. Continue taking progesterone if this has been prescribed for you, but contact your fertility unit if you are taking HCG injections as these make OHSS worse.

Contact your fertility unit and tell them about your symptoms. They will give you advice over the telephone and arrange to see you. If you have severe pain or breathlessness you need to be seen urgently. Your unit should have 24-hour contact numbers so that you can speak to an experienced member of staff. In an emergency, go to the accident and emergency department of your local hospital. Take with you any information you have about your treatment, such as the fertility drug schedule and the unit's information leaflet about OHSS—if you don't have one, take this book!

What treatment is available?

Your fertility unit should have a protocol for treatment of OHSS which should be available to local accident and emergency departments and gynaecology departments. Guidelines are also published by the Royal College of Obstetricians and Gynaecologists and are freely available on the Internet (www.rcog.org.uk).

The first step is to assess how bad the condition is. After examining your abdomen, an ultrasound scan will show how large your ovaries are and whether there is a build-up of fluid. A blood test will show whether the blood is concentrated (a sign of dehydration) and check the function of the kidneys and liver.

Most women with mild or moderate OHSS can stay at home, but you may need to be seen frequently in the unit (every 2 or 3 days) for monitoring until the illness improves. Tablets can be prescribed to relieve pain and sickness.

If the OHSS is getting worse, you will need to be admitted to hospital. Monitoring may include your weight, waist measurement, and amount of urine passed each day. Fluid can be given through a drip if you cannot drink enough, and effective medicines can be prescribed for sickness and pain. To prevent blood clots you will be given 'airline stockings' to wear and may have a daily injection of an anti-clotting drug.

It is important to be seen by a gynaecologist because a few other conditions can mimic OHSS (twisted ovary, bleeding ovarian cyst, pelvic infection, ectopic pregnancy) and these need to be identified, as they need different treatment.

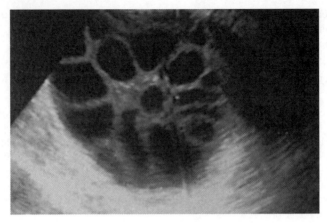

Figure 15.1 Ultrasound scan of enlarged ovary and excess fluid in severe OHSS.

Severe hyperstimulation

If OHSS is severe, you definitely need to be in hospital. If there are signs of fluid around the lungs, you will have a chest X-ray or scan to show this. Sometimes the fluid building up in the abdomen needs to be drained. This is done using a needle which is watched on an ultrasound scan, rather like an egg collection procedure, but usually done through the skin of the abdomen using local anaesthetic. This is very effective in relieving pain and breathlessness. Rarely, drainage of fluid from the chest and a scan of the heart (echocardiogram) will be needed as well. A drip and bladder catheter will monitor fluid in and out of the body. The intensive care unit may be the best place to do this.

Are there long-term effects?

OHSS always gets better, although it may take several weeks. There are no known long-term effects. Women who have had OHSS will be at risk of the same thing happening again if they have another treatment cycle. Changing the drug regime might lessen the risk. If you attend a different fertility unit in future, it is important to tell them about OHSS.

Hyperstimulation and pregnancy

Women who suffer from severe OHSS are often pregnant. Probably the early hormone changes of pregnancy worsen the condition by stimulating the ovaries. OHSS tends to begin later in the treatment cycle and last longer in women who are pregnant.

There is no evidence that OHSS causes any abnormalities in pregnancy, and the pregnancy should continue normally.

All medicines used in treating OHSS are chosen to be safe if you are pregnant.

Case study

Denise had polycystic ovary syndrome. She and her partner James had had IVF and 24 eggs had been collected. Two embryos were replaced. They were delighted, but Denise started to feel unwell, with bloating and nausea, on the third day after egg collection. By the sixth day, she was so sick that she couldn't keep any liquids down and was admitted to hospital. She was prescribed a drip, painkillers, anti-clotting stockings, and injections. Her HCG injections were changed to progesterone suppositories. She was very bloated. Ultrasound scan showed that this was due to fluid collected in her tummy. After six days in hospital, she still felt awful, but the compensation was a positive pregnancy test. After 12 days in hospital, she was finally well enough to go home.

16

Preimplantation genetic tests

➔ Key points

◆ Preimplantation genetic diagnosis (PGD) requires IVF, and is a test for inherited conditions carried out on the embryo.

◆ Alternatives to PGD include prenatal diagnosis (at 10–16 weeks of pregnancy) or egg/sperm donation.

◆ Pre-implantation genetic screening (PGS) tests embryos for common chromosome abnormalities.

◆ The aim of PGS is to select healthy embryos for transfer to the womb. However, PGS has not been shown to improve IVF pregnancy rates.

Preimplantation genetic screening (PGS) is a new method of embryo screening increasingly used in older women undergoing IVF to screen for Down syndrome and chromosomal abnormalities.

Preimplantation genetic diagnosis (PGD) is a test developed to help couples who are at risk of passing on an inherited disease to have a healthy family. It is carried out on embryos and needs IVF first (see Chapter 14). These couples have normal fertility and would conceive naturally, but choose to undergo IVF in order to have PGD. PGD tests for a particular inherited disease.

Preimplantation genetic diagnosis is complicated and some of the terminology is scientific. Depending on how much information you need, the science sections have been placed into boxes for easy reading (or to leave out!). However, if you are undergoing PGD, you will want as much information as possible and understanding the scientific terms is important.

Preimplantation genetic diagnosis can help:

◆ couples who have a family history of a serious inherited problem

◆ couples who have had an affected baby

◆ couples with a previous history of repeated miscarriages due to a chromosomal problem.

The alternative to preimplantation genetic diagnosis is prenatal diagnosis (amniocentesis or chorionic villus sampling) between 10 and 16 weeks of pregnancy to find out if the baby is affected. Other options are egg or sperm donation.

Preimplantation genetic diagnosis involves IVF and testing a single cell from the embryo. Although many PGD couples are fertile, routine IVF procedures are required so that embryos are generated outside the body for biopsy and PGD. Unaffected embryos can be transferred into the womb.

The most common method of PGD is cleavage stage biopsy. This involves testing one or two cells (blastomeres) from an embryo containing six to eight cells (a six- to eight-cell embryo).

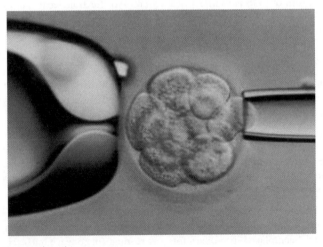

Figure 16.1 Embryo biopsy.

IVF/ICSI	is needed to create embryos for testing
↓	
Diagnostic work-up	each test is specifically developed for the particular inherited problem
↓	

Healthy embryos are transferred back to the womb

What is DNA? What is a gene? What is a chromosome?

The human body is made up of more than 100 million cells. Each cell has a different job to do: muscle cells, nerve cells, blood cells. Each cell contains the instructions coded in the form of a chemical called deoxyribonucleic acid (DNA). DNA is organized into genes that are arranged on thread-like structures called chromosomes. Every chromosome contains thousands of genes, each with enough information for the production of one protein. This protein may determine eye or hair colour, for example.

Every body cell contains 46 chromosomes arranged in 23 pairs. One of each pair comes from the mother and one from the father. Eggs and sperm have only half that number, so that when an egg is fertilized, the new individual is assured of having the correct number of chromosomes.

At the moment of fertilization, the genes start giving instructions for the development of a new human being. The father's chromosomes are responsible for sex determination. One pair of his chromosomes are called X or Y, depending on their shape. In women, both the chromosomes in the pair are X, but in men there is one X and one Y. If an X-containing sperm fertilizes an X egg, the baby will be a girl, but if a Y sperm fertilizes the egg, then the baby will be a boy.

Different types of test are needed to detect different types of inherited problem

Polymerase chain reaction (PCR)

PCR involves duplicating the genetic material in the cell millions of times. There is then enough to test. It is used for the diagnosis of single-gene defects, such as cystic fibrosis, or the triplet repeat disorders such as myotonic dystrophy.

If a sperm embedded in the wall of the egg is dislodged during the test, this genetic material will also be duplicated and the accuracy of the result can be affected. Therefore the ICSI technique (intracytoplasmic sperm injection) is

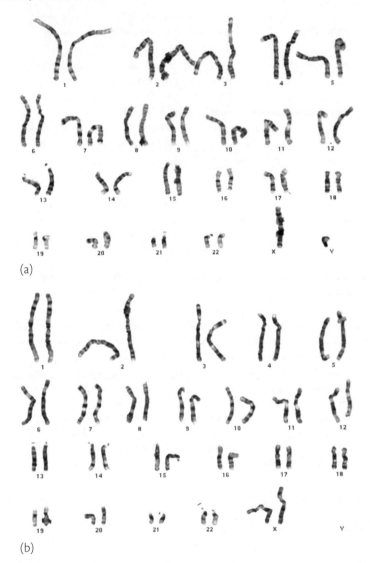

Figure 16.2 Chromosomes: (a) normal male pattern with one X chromosome and one Y chromosome; (b) normal female pattern with two X chromosomes.

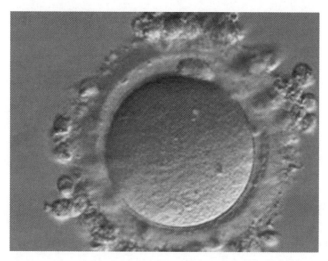

Figure 16.3 An egg surrounded by cumulus cells from the ovary. These cells can affect the accuracy of testing because they are from the mother, not the embryo.

used to inject a single sperm into the oocyte, so that extra sperm do not become embedded in the wall of the egg (see Chapter 14).

Fluorescent *in situ* hybridization (FISH)

FISH involves labelling the genetic material for a particular abnormality. It is used to analyse the presence or absence of a chromosome or part of a chromosome. This can be for sexing by probes for the X and Y chromosomes and for PGD of chromosome abnormalities, such as translocations, by probes for the chromosomes involved in the specific translocation.

Cumulus cells from the mother surround the embryo and may also be labelled, affecting the accuracy. In addition, not all the cells of an embryo are the same (mosaicism), and so the cell tested may not be representative of the whole. Usually, any embryos remaining after transfer following PGD are used to confirm the diagnosis.

Inherited problems that can be diagnosed by PGD

Inherited problems that can be diagnosed by PGD are listed in the boxes. The list is changing all the time as new tests develop.

Dominant disorders

- Marfan syndrome
- Familial adenomatous polyposis coli
- Charcot–Marie–Tooth disease (type 1A)
- Osteogenesis imperfecta
- Crouzon syndrome
- Neurofibromatosis type 2
- Li–Fraumeni syndrome

Single-gene defects (dominant and recessive)

- Cystic fibrosis (various mutations)
- Tay–Sachs disease
- Beta-thalassaemia
- Sickle cell anaemia
- Rhesus blood typing
- Spinal muscular atrophy
- Adrenogenital syndrome
- Congenital adrenal hyperplasia
- Plakophilin-1 (PKP1)
- Medium-chain acyl CoA dehydrogenase deficiency

Triplet repeat disorders

- Myotonic dystrophy
- Huntington's disease
- Fragile X syndrome

Sexing for X-linked disease

- Lesch–Nyhan syndrome
- Duchenne muscular dystrophy
- Charcot–Marie–Tooth disease
- Retinitis pigmentosa
- Ornithine transcarbamylase deficiency

Clinical aspects of preimplantation genetic diagnosis

Before couples are referred for preimplantation genetic diagnosis, they have usually already had genetic counselling. It is important to explain IVF treatment and PGD testing. If a couple want to go ahead with preimplantation genetic diagnosis, the next step is development of the test (diagnostic work-up). Apart from sexing the embryo for X-linked disease, all other preimplantation genetic diagnostic tests involve developing a test specifically for the couple. This stage can take several months or more. In the UK, all preimplantation genetic diagnostic tests need to be approved by the Human Fertilisation and Embryology Authority (HFEA), which licences all IVF and PGD procedures, and application must be made before any treatment is commenced.

When this stage is complete, couples require a full IVF and PGD consultation, including gynaecological and fertility tests routine to IVF procedures (such as sperm count, hormone tests, examination of the uterus, trial embryo transfer). For PGD patients, especially those carrying fragile X syndrome, a test of ovarian reserve is recommended. This is to make sure that the ovary can respond to the fertility drugs to produce additional eggs.

PGD is identical to regular IVF except that ovarian stimulation aims to maximize the number of eggs retrieved. This increases the risk of ovarian hyperstimulation (see Chapter 15). For PGD to be successful, at least nine eggs are needed in order to have enough embryos to test and enough good-quality unaffected embryos to replace. In some cycles, all embryos will be affected and no embryos will be available for replacement. In PGD, the diagnosis is made from one or two cells. Because of the problems of single-cell diagnosis and mosaicism, it is recommended that pregnant women undergo prenatal diagnosis, but in practice only 50 per cent of patients opt for this.

The European Society of Human Reproduction and Endocrinology (ESHRE) Preimplantation Genetic Diagnosis Consortium was set up in 1997. It aims to study all aspects of PGD, allow the sharing of information about PGD, to collect information about accuracy, reliability and effectiveness, and follow-up of pregnancies and children born after preimplantation genetic testing.

The sixth report of the ESHRE PGD Consortium related to cycles collected for the calendar year 2003 and follow-up of the pregnancies and babies born up to October 2004. Fifty centres participated, reporting on 2868 cycles, 501 pregnancies, and 373 babies born. The PGD Consortium data include cycles for preimplantation genetic diagnosis, preimplantation genetic screening, and cycles for social sexing. The data do not account for all PGD cycles. Although some of the patients were fertile, the pregnancy rate for preimplantation was low (15 per cent per egg retrieval or 24 per cent per embryo transfer), probably because of the reduction in the number of embryos that are suitable for transfer.

The number of different types of disease diagnosed by PGD has remained low because of the technical nature of the test.

Success rates for preimplantation genetic diagnosis

◆ One in seven (15%) per egg retrieval

◆ One in four (24%) per embryo transfer

Not every cycle of treatment will produce embryos suitable for transfer.

Preimplantation genetic screening (PGS)

Preimplantation screening is a new technique for embryo screening. It is increasingly used by older women going through IVF, by couples who have experienced repeated IVF failure because their embryos do not implant in the womb, and by couples who have experienced recurrent miscarriages. Embryos can be screened for Down syndrome and abnormalities of chromosomes 13,16, 18, and 20 before they are replaced in the womb. This should improve the success rate of treatment by selecting only healthy embryos and reduce the risk of miscarriage, but is not yet proven. Following IVF (see Chapter 14), the developing embryo is checked by taking a single cell or two cells for genetic analysis. The cells are examined for the number of chromosomes present using specially designed 'probes' that identify the most common abnormalities such as an extra chromosome 21, which causes Down syndrome. Only embryos with normal chromosome results are put back into the woman's body. There are drawbacks to this technique. For example, the cell studied may not be identical to the rest of the embryo, not all chromosomes can be checked, and there are safety concerns that removing cells from an embryo might affect later development.

The sixth report of the ESHRE PGD Consortium reported 2950 cycles for preimplantation genetic screening. Of these, 702 had a positive pregnancy test. The clinical pregnancy rate was 17 per cent per egg collection or 24 per cent per embryo transfer.

Success rates for preimplantation genetic screening

◆ One in six (17%) per egg retrieval

◆ One in four (24%) per embryo transfer

The future

The future of preimplantation genetic diagnosis is to develop better and more accurate tests. This can be achieved by basic DNA fingerprinting to ensure that the DNA analysed is embryonic and techniques such as multiplex PCR, which can be employed to maximize the information obtained from a single cell. A technique called 'comparative genomic hybridization' allows assessment of all the cell's chromosomes at once. This can be applied to eggs before they are fertilized, rather than creating and testing embryos. The time taken for the procedure is too long for clinical PGD but future developments involving DNA chip technology could eventually allow monitoring of all IVF embryos for chromosome status. Avoiding the transfer of those embryos with lethal abnormalities could lead to an improvement in the implantation rate per embryo transferred and reduce the risk of multiple pregnancies.

17

Sperm donation (donor insemination)

➡ Key points

- Sperm donation (donor insemination) is an option for couples if the man is unable to produce sperm, if the numbers of sperm are too low to achieve a pregnancy, or if there is a very high risk of passing on a serious inherited disease.

- Women who do not have a male partner can also be treated with donor insemination.

- About 3000 women in the UK are currently undergoing donor insemination treatment; 700–800 babies are born each year in the UK as a result of sperm donation.

- The success rate for donor insemination in the UK is 14 per cent per month for women aged less than 35; for women aged 40 and over, the success rate is 5 per cent per month.

- Following a change in UK law in 2005, children now have the right to access their genetic origin and find out the identity of their donor when they reach the age of 18.

When is donor insemination needed?

Donor insemination is offered to couples if the man is unable to make sperm, or the numbers of sperm are so low that they cannot achieve a pregnancy.

Over the last 10 years, the development of ICSI, which allows a single sperm to be injected into an egg (see Chapter 14), has allowed many men with very low sperm counts to father children by IVF, and as a result fewer couples are choosing donor insemination. However, some couples prefer donor insemination if the woman has no fertility problems and they want to avoid IVF.

If the semen contains no sperm, this could be because of a blockage in the tubes that carry sperm out of the testicles. If so, it may still be possible to collect sperm from the testicles with a small surgical procedure and use it for ICSI (more details are given in chapter 10). Couples may need to weigh up the success rate, availability, and cost of having these sperm extraction techniques with ICSI compared with donor insemination.

If a man is not producing any sperm from the testicles, the only treatment option for the couple is donor insemination.

Donor sperm may also be used if there is a very high risk of passing on a serious inherited disease. A possible alternative treatment for some couples is IVF with testing of embryos before they are put into the womb (see Chapter 16).

Women who do not have a male partner can also be treated with donor insemination. Increasing numbers of single women and lesbian couples are seeking treatment.

Is treatment available?

In the latest national figures published in the UK, almost 3000 women were going through donor insemination treatment, about a third of whom were women without a male partner. A total of 700–800 babies are born each year.

The majority of these treatments are carried out in the private sector. NHS funding for donor insemination is not available in all areas. Policy varies between different primary care trusts, and you should approach your GP or local NHS fertility unit for advice. At present, not all clinics offer treatment to same-sex couples or single women.

There is a national shortage of sperm donors and so there may be waiting lists for treatment, even in the private sector. It is worth approaching two or three clinics to ask about waiting times.

Because of the shortage of donors from some ethnic groups, it may be very difficult for some couples to obtain treatment.

Is it necessary to use a clinic?

Home treatment with donor insemination has been practised successfully, particularly in the gay community. However, this cannot be recommended. It is not as safe as treatment in a licensed clinic, where all donors are screened for inherited disease and viral infections. There may be a risk of infection when using fresh sperm from an unscreened donor. Also, the semen samples have not been checked for quality, so treatment may be ineffective. The legal position is less clear, especially with a known donor who might be able to make a claim on the child.

There are Internet services which provide fresh sperm samples for home insemination, but again you do not have all the safeguards of using a licensed clinic.

Who are the donors?

Sperm donors are volunteers. Fertility clinics may recruit their own donors or purchase sperm from banks in the UK or overseas. There is also a national organization, the National Gamete Donation Trust, which has been set up to raise awareness and increase recruitment of donors. Traditionally, donors tended to be college students, but now the profile of donors is changing and some are men with their own families who want to help others.

Donors must be healthy men of normal fertility. They cannot be aged over 45 or less than 19. They undergo medical screening and fertility testing before being accepted as donors (see below: 'Is treatment safe?')

Donors in the UK are not paid, but they receive a small amount of money to cover expenses for travel or loss of earnings.

All donors attending licensed clinics receive counselling to make sure that they understand the implications of sperm donation and are aware of their rights, and the rights of the prospective parents and the children who may be born. The removal of anonymity from donors, which occurred in the UK in 2005, means that children have the right to access their genetic origin and find out the identity of their donor. Donors agree that their details will be held on a register and can be released to their donor-conceived children who are aged 18 or over.

Will I know who the donor is?

The great majority of sperm donation in the UK is anonymous to the recipient. The couple receiving treatment do not meet the donor or know his name. Neither does the donor have any access to the couple being treated. A code is used to identify the donor in the clinic records.

The clinic can give 'non-identifying information' to the couple receiving treatment. This may include the donor's ethnic background, hair and eye colour, height, and weight. Donors are also encouraged to write a 'pen portrait' describing their personality and interests, for example if they are musical or sporty. These details can be available to the child later.

Some couples choose to use a known donor, either a friend or a family member related to the husband. This is acceptable if everyone agrees. It is important to look at all the implications, particularly how the donor might be involved with the future child.

Will the baby look like me?

Your clinic will record your physical characteristics (your hair and skin colour etc.) and will match the donor to you and your partner as closely as possible. The clinic will be able to tell you the physical characteristics of the donors available. Of course, matching does not guarantee that your baby will look like you. Not all children conceived naturally look like their parents!

Is the treatment safe? (Donor screening)

Donors undergo detailed screening before being accepted. They must not have any significant medical disease, disability, or family history of disease that could be inherited. With their permission, their GP is contacted to confirm that there is no medical history that could affect their donation.

Donors are all screened for sexually transmitted diseases, and they have blood tests for viral infections including HIV (the AIDS virus), hepatitis B, and hepatitis C. All semen samples are frozen and kept in quarantine until the donor has completed follow-up tests; this makes sure that he was not incubating any viral infection at the time of donation. There has not been any case of transmission of HIV through donor insemination under UK regulations.

Donors are also screened for CMV (cytomegalovirus). This is a common viral infection which causes a flu-like illness. It can be harmful in pregnant women because it can pass to the baby. The possibility of CMV infection being transmitted in semen is controversial as there is no definite proof of this, but, as a safeguard, CMV-negative women (i.e. those without immunity to CMV) are only treated with CMV-negative donors.

Is the treatment effective? (Success rates)

The success rate for donor insemination in the UK is 14 per cent per month for women aged under 35. This falls to 5 per cent per month for women of 40 and over. These figures sound low compared with IVF, but insemination is a simple treatment which can be repeated month after month, and 30–50 per cent of couples will be pregnant after 6 months.

If insemination is not successful, you may go on to have IVF with donor sperm.

Is treatment confidential?

Your treatment is confidential. Under the Human Fertilization and Embryology Act 1990, it is a criminal offence for the clinic to reveal confidential information such as the identity of the donor. Information can only be given out with your consent.

It is sensible to inform your GP. You may need to involve him/her in your treatment; moreover, he/she will be looking after you and your family in the long term and should be aware of all your medical treatment. Medical information may also be needed by your consultant, or by staff treating you in an emergency.

The clinic will ask you to give consent to disclosure by signing a form. Some couples decide to limit the information given out, so that correspondence about their treatment does not mention the use of donor sperm. As well as medical disclosure, the clinic may need to use the information about your treatment for audit (e.g. calculating their success rates) and for financial accounts. Every cycle of treatment in the UK is recorded by the HFEA, which levies a fee on the clinics to cover its work of regulation and inspection.

Are any tests needed beforehand?

Certain tests are needed before treatment (see Chapter 7 for screening tests needed before fertility treatment). Women should check that they are immune to rubella and up to date with cervical smear testing before pregnancy. Chlamydia screening should be done before insemination; swabs from the vagina and cervix will make sure that there is no infection that could be worsened by the insemination procedures. In the UK, all couples undergoing treatment are tested for HIV and hepatitis infection. Clinics also screen women for CMV.

To make sure that insemination treatment will be effective, some tests are done to check the woman's fertility. Ovulation is usually confirmed with a timed blood test for progesterone. The womb and ovaries are checked with an ultrasound scan, and this may be done with a second blood test for ovarian function. The Fallopian tubes must be open. This can be checked in several ways. The most common test is an X-ray called a hysterosalpingogram (HSG) which passes dye through the cervix into the womb and tubes so that an X-ray pictures can be taken. Some clinics perform a similar test using ultrasound which is called HyCoSy. If a problem is suspected then a laparoscopy test may be needed. All these tests are described in more detail in Chapter 7.

How is the treatment carried out?

Intra-cervical insemination is the simplest form of treatment. The donor semen is thawed in the laboratory and its quality checked under the microscope. It is drawn up with a syringe into a fine tube. Using an instrument to see the cervix, the nurse or doctor places the semen into the external opening of the cervix. The woman rests for short time before going home.

Timing of the insemination is crucial. It must be done at the time of ovulation, and the woman will be asked to check the day of ovulation by using home urine tests for the LH surge (see Chapter 7). Sometimes two treatments are given on successive days.

Intra-cervical insemination is not commonly performed nowadays since better success rates are achieved with intra-uterine insemination.

In intra-uterine insemination the donor semen sample is thawed and prepared in the laboratory to concentrate the sperm, resulting in a small volume (half a millilitre) of fertile sperm that is drawn up into a very fine tube and passed through the cervix. The sample is then released into the womb so that the sperm are flushed up the Fallopian tubes.

Fertility drugs are often used to improve the chance of success, especially if the woman is not ovulating regularly. Even for women who ovulate normally, the use of fertility drugs will stimulate ovulation and may cause the release of more than one egg (see Chapter 11). This improves success rates but also carries a risk of multiple pregnancy. Clomifene, which is taken as a tablet, is the most commonly used fertility drug. Gonadotrophin injections can also be used.

What happens if it doesn't work?

Donor insemination treatment should be repeated for several months. Like natural conception, given time, more and more couples will become pregnant. Usually it is worth trying for at least 6 months.

IVF with donor sperm is sometimes needed if the simpler forms of treatment have not succeeded. It may also be advised if the woman has a significant fertility problem, such as damaged tubes, as insemination is not likely to work.

What happens if I become pregnant?

Your pregnancy test will be positive 2 weeks after the insemination procedure. The fertility clinic will offer you an ultrasound scan in early pregnancy. This is usually done at 7 weeks gestation (5 weeks from insemination). At this stage an embryo and heartbeat can usually be seen, and multiple pregnancy can be detected. Ectopic (tubal) pregnancy is uncommon but may be diagnosed.

You will need to decide, with advice from your clinic and your GP, where you will have the baby. Your GP usually refers you to the antenatal clinic and you will be seen there at 12 weeks of pregnancy (see Chapter 24 for advice in early pregnancy).

There are no particular risks in pregnancy related to donor insemination. As explained above, it is up to you whether you tell the midwife and doctor looking after you that the pregnancy was conceived with donor sperm.

What do we put on the birth certificate?

In British law, a woman giving birth is the legal mother. If you and your male partner have been treated together as a couple at a licensed clinic in the UK, you are the legal parents and so your names should be put on the birth certificate.

As the law stands at present, if you are a single woman being treated without a partner, the child will have no legal father.

'Parental responsibility'

When a child is born to a married couple, they both automatically have rights and duties towards the child which are termed 'parental responsibility'. This is defined by law (the Children's Act 1989 in England and Wales, and similar provisions in Scotland and Northern Ireland). Where an unmarried couple are being treated, the male partner will not automatically have 'parental responsibility' and it is recommended that unmarried couples should seek legal advice about the male partner's rights and responsibilities towards the child. In future the Act may be amended so that an unmarried father who registers the child's birth jointly with the mother will acquire parental responsibility.

The donor has no parental rights or legal responsibilities towards the child, as long as treatment was carried out through a licensed clinic in the UK.

Should I tell my child?

Parents are advised to be honest with their children. In the past, many parents of donor-conceived children kept this a secret. They worried that the father's position in the family would be threatened if it were known that he was not the genetic father. However, times have changed and there should be no stigma attached to fertility treatment. Children need to understand their origins, and it is much better for them to absorb this knowledge as they grow up rather than discover it later, which can occur as a result of medical tests or a traumatic disclosure during a family argument.

It may not be easy to approach telling your child. Your clinic counsellor can be very helpful, and you may be able to contact him or her even though your treatment was some time ago. There are also patient organizations which can support you with telephone helplines and publications (see 'Useful addresses').

What could my child find out?

The clinic treating you can provide you with 'non-identifying information' such as the donor's ethnic background, hair and eye colour, height, and weight. The donor may also have written a 'pen portrait' describing himself, or a message to the child.

When children reach the age of 18, they can apply to the HFEA for confirmation that they were born following donor treatment. Following a change in the law from April 2005, they are legally entitled to obtain details of the identity of their genetic parent. The HFEA maintains a register of all UK donors. The register is also used to ensure that donor-conceived children do not accidentally marry someone related to them.

We want to have more than one child

If sperm is still available from the same donor, you can use it to have another child who will be a genetic brother or sister. You can ask the clinic to reserve samples for you to use in the future; there may be a fee for this. Sperm can be frozen and stored for up to 10 years.

Because of the shortage of sperm donors, one donor may be used in the treatment of several women. Thus your donor-conceived children may have genetic half-brothers and half-sisters. In the UK, the use of samples from one donor is limited to no more than 10 births. Even if the limit of 10 births from one donor has been reached, it is still possible for the same donor to be used for sibling pregnancies, i.e. to create 10 families.

Making a decision on donor treatment

Even with all the information from your doctor and from this book, you may still find it hard to make a decision on treatment with donor sperm. It can be difficult for couples who have gone through infertility investigations to come to terms with the results, and to accept that they will not be able to have genetic children. Some people have religious or ethical concerns about gamete donation. Many have anxieties about how they will feel towards the child, whether they should tell their family, and how their own parents might react.

It is an important decision and will have long-term consequences, and so you need to take enough time to discuss it with your partner, and perhaps with family or friends. Professional help from a fertility counsellor can be invaluable, and your clinic will offer this. You may also want to contact a patient support group (see 'Useful addresses') to see how others have coped with the same situation.

18

Egg donation

Why is egg donation needed?

Donor eggs are needed when a woman's ovaries no longer contain eggs, following an early menopause, or the eggs she has are poor quality. Early menopause can be caused by surgery on the ovaries, by chemotherapy treatment for cancer, or by medical conditions such as Turner syndrome (a genetic condition in which the ovaries do not fully develop). It often comes out of the blue; premature menopause affects one woman in 100 below the age of 40. Poor egg quality is usually found in older women, and is often diagnosed after tests for miscarriage or infertility, perhaps after several unsuccessful IVF attempts. Egg donation is also sometimes used by women who carry a serious inherited disorder so that they do not pass it on to their children.

Who donates the eggs?

Donors are volunteers. Most egg donors are not related or known to the woman receiving the eggs. Donors may be recruited by advertisements, which may be placed by clinics or by couples seeking treatment. Some donors contact clinics because they have seen a magazine or newspaper article or a TV programme about egg donation. Others volunteer because they know someone who is going through fertility treatment.

In the UK some clinics offer 'egg sharing'. This means that healthy women who are going through IVF treatment may give away some of their eggs, while keeping the rest for their own use. Usually the couple receiving the eggs will cover the costs of the donor's IVF treatment.

It is also possible for a couple to use a known donor who is a relative or friend, for example the woman's sister. This may be preferable for some families because the child will be genetically related as closely as possible to the mother. They may also feel more comfortable with a known donor than an anonymous stranger. However, it is very important to talk through all the implications. For example, how does the donor's partner feel? How will the donor feel in the future? What if she never has children of her own? Will the donor be involved in the child's upbringing?

Are donors paid?

In the UK, where treatment is regulated by the HFEA, donation is altruistic and donors cannot be paid. Expenses can be reimbursed, for example to cover the cost of travelling to the clinic, costs of childcare, or loss of earnings (to an upper limit currently set at £250). Outside the UK, regulations vary and in some countries donors are paid quite substantial amounts.

Is egg donation available?

There is a severe shortage of egg donors in the UK. Waiting lists can vary widely between clinics and can be 2 years or more, so it is worth contacting several clinics to enquire about waiting times and their strategies to recruit donors. It is possible to have your name on more than one list (although you should be open with the clinics if you intend to do this, and inform them if you have treatment elsewhere, so that other patients are not disadvantaged).

You may want to advertise to recruit a donor, and most clinics will help you with this. For example, they may have examples of advertisements that have previously been successful, or posters that you could put up. The poster will have your reference number, so that you remain anonymous, and the clinic telephone number.

If you are able to introduce a donor, but do not want to use her eggs yourself (for example, if a friend of yours volunteers to help), then a 'cross-over' system can benefit everyone—your friend donates anonymously to another couple, and in exchange you receive priority on the waiting list for the next suitable donor.

Egg donation is not usually funded by the NHS. Policy on NHS funding varies between different areas and you should approach your primary care trust or health board, or ask your GP or local fertility clinic for advice. Some authorities will fund egg donation on an individual basis, particularly if there are clear medical reasons for infertility, such as childhood cancer treatment. NHS funding is not given to women aged over 40.

Egg donation is available in other countries, and an increasing number of British couples are going abroad for treatment. The most common destination in Europe is Spain; treatment is also easily available (although expensive) in the USA, and clinics in other counties have a growing British clientele. However, couples seeking treatment overseas need to do careful research and consider possible risks. The laws governing treatment may be different, laboratory regulation and inspection may not be as strict, and record keeping may not be as detailed. Donors might be attracted by the offer of payment; there are concerns that recruitment of donors from economically deprived communities is not really 'voluntary' donation. In most counties donation is anonymous and it will not be possible for the child to trace the donor in future years.

Some British clinics have now set up links with clinics abroad, so that couples can have treatment organized in the UK and fly out to have the embryo transfer in the satellite clinic.

How are egg donors tested?

Donors must be healthy women with enough eggs to donate. In the UK, donors should be younger than 36 except in exceptional circumstances (such as sister-to-sister donation). Donors will have their ovarian function checked with ultrasound scanning and a hormone blood test before starting treatment, and will not be able to donate if they do not produce enough eggs.

A detailed medical history is taken from the donor, and any significant medical problems, such as diabetes, will exclude her from donating. A family history is also taken, to see whether there is any hereditary disease that might be passed on. Donors are also tested with a chromosome analysis and screened to see if they carry any of the most common genetic diseases: cystic fibrosis in Caucasians, sickle cell disease in African Caribbeans, and thalassaemia in Mediterranean and South Asian donors.

Donors are screened for virus infections that might be passed on through body fluids: HIV, hepatitis B, hepatitis C, and CMV (see Chapter 17). They are also screened for sexually transmitted infection.

Will I know the donor's identity?

In the UK, the donor's identity is protected by law. Unless you are using a known donor whom you have introduced to the clinic, you will not be told the identity of your donor. Her name will not appear in your medical notes, but a code number is used. The clinic keeps separate records for donors, and, if necessary, the donor can be traced through the code.

Can my child learn the donor's identity?

Yes. In the UK all donors are registered with the HFEA. Following a change in the law in 2005, it is possible for people born from egg donation (and sperm and embryo donation) to apply to the register when they are aged 18 to confirm that their birth resulted from donation and to obtain details of the donor's identity. They may also ask the registry to check that they are not related to the person they intend to marry.

Can the donor contact me or my child?

No, unless you are using a known donor. Your treatment is confidential and the donor is not told your identity. The clinic is allowed to inform her whether or not her donation has been successful, if she wishes to know, and donors may feel a great sense of achievement. However, she will not be able to obtain your identity or contact your child, and she has no legal rights or any responsibilities towards your child,

Is my treatment confidential?

Yes, your treatment is confidential and by law the clinic can only disclose information with your consent. You will be asked to give consent by signing a form which allows the clinic to inform your GP and other relevant health professionals (for example, to refer you to hospital in an emergency). In addition to medical disclosure, the clinic may need to use the information about your treatment for audit (e.g. calculating their success rates) and for financial accounts.

You can decide to restrict the information given out, so that correspondence about your treatment does not mention the use of donor eggs. If you become pregnant, it is advisable to inform the doctor and midwife looking after you, because it may affect your care, particularly if you are offered antenatal tests for Down syndrome (the risk of Down syndrome relates not to your age but to the age of the egg donor).

Counselling

With so much to consider, it can be a very difficult decision to go ahead with treatment with donated eggs. It is a decision which could have lifelong implications, and the help of a professional fertility counsellor can be very valuable. The discovery that you will not be able to get pregnant with your own eggs can be a devastating blow, and again a counsellor may help you to handle this and support you through treatment. A counsellor will be available at your clinic. There are also several patient organizations which can provide information and support (see 'Useful addresses'), and you may be able to get in touch with other couples who have been in your situation.

Egg donors also need to consider the implications carefully. They need to be aware of what the medical treatment will involve and possible risks, but it is just as important to consider the psychological aspects. Donors must be aware that their identity can be revealed in future, and they could be contacted by the children born from their donation. Egg sharers need to consider how they might feel if their own treatment does not work but the recipient is successful, so that another couple will be bringing up a child that is genetically theirs. Donors have the right to withdraw from the process at any time until the embryos are transferred to the recipient.

The HFEA information leaflet *Donating sperm, eggs or embryos* is very useful for anyone considering becoming a donor and is available on the HFEA website (www.hfea.gov.uk).

What tests will I need before treatment?

Before treatment, you and your partner will need tests for viral infections (HIV, hepatitis B, and hepatitis C), and the female partner will need tests for CMV and rubella. The male partner will need to have a semen analysis.

The woman will need a check of the womb using ultrasound (or sometimes an X-ray or hysteroscopy). Some clinics will do a 'mock embryo transfer' to make sure that this will be an easy procedure on the actual day of transfer. You may be advised to have a 'dummy run' by taking hormone supplements for 2–3 weeks with ultrasound checks on the womb; this is particularly useful if you have had early menopause from radiotherapy to the abdomen or pelvic area.

If there is any medical history which could affect pregnancy, this should be dealt with before treatment. For example, some women with early menopause following cancer treatment may have had chemotherapy that can also damage the heart or kidneys. Women with Turner syndrome should have a full medical review before pregnancy, as they might be at risk of high blood pressure and diabetes, and death from serious cardiac complications has been reported.

What does the treatment involve?

The woman receiving the eggs has simpler treatment than the donor! She takes hormone supplements to prepare the womb for embryo transfer while the donor is going through ovarian stimulation and egg collection.

The menstrual cycles of the donor and recipient need to be lined up so that fresh embryos can be transferred. If the recipient is already on HRT, it is easy to adjust the cycle by a few days. If both women have natural cycles, it is often done by taking one packet of the Pill, and blocking the natural cycle with GnRH analogue (as described in Chapter 14).

The recipient will need to take oestrogen tablets to build up the womb lining. This takes about 2 weeks, and is monitored by ultrasound scan. Meanwhile the donor receives daily injections to stimulate her ovaries to make plenty of mature eggs. (This is described in more detail in Chapter 14.) On the day of egg collection, the recipient's husband will be asked to attend clinic to provide a fresh sperm sample to fertilize the donated eggs. The oestrogen treatment continues and progesterone is added to mature the womb lining. Progesterone can be given as injections or vaginal tablets. A few days later, when the embryos are ready, the couple will attend clinic for embryo transfer.

One or two embryos will be drawn up into a fine tube and passed through the vagina into the womb, where they are released. Over the next few days the embryos may develop and stick to the wall of the womb. Hormone supplements need to be continued for at least 2 weeks until a pregnancy test is done. If positive, treatment needs to be continued to support the pregnancy for the first few weeks. It is usually tapered off and stopped at 12 weeks. By then, the pregnancy is self-supporting and produces its own hormones from the placenta.

Are there any risks?

There are minimal risks to the woman receiving the eggs. Side effects from hormone supplements are unlikely (although progesterone injections can be painful); a very rare complication is thrombosis. There are potential risks in pregnancy, as mentioned earlier; women having egg donation are often older than other patients and more prone to pregnancy complications.

The donor has a small risk of ovarian hyperstimulation following fertility drug treatment (see Chapter 15) or infection or bleeding as a result of the egg collection procedure. She may have lower abdominal discomfort for a few days around the time of egg retrieval. During the donation cycle, the donor should use barrier contraception or avoid intercourse as she might become pregnant.

Complications are unlikely, but donors who are volunteering to go through medical procedures need to know any possible risks. There should be no long-term effects. The donor's fertility should not be affected.

Is egg donation successful?

Egg donation is the most successful type of IVF treatment. Success rates are usually 30–35 per cent or more per embryo transfer. Pregnancy rates are better for egg recipients than for women having IVF with their own eggs, probably because egg donors are fertile young women and the recipient's womb lining is carefully prepared.

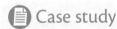 Case study

June was 26 when her periods became erratic: she had none for 6 months at a time, and eventually they stopped completely. She saw her GP because she was waking at night with hot sweats. The GP took a blood test for hormone levels and said that it showed an early menopause; he had never seen this happen to anyone so young and arranged for her to see a specialist.

June's real concern was that she wanted children. The specialist said that this was extremely unlikely, as she had had no periods for 3 years. He started her on HRT, which cured her night sweats.

June contacted the doctor again when she got engaged to Ed. They went together to the fertility clinic and talked about egg donation. June had a younger sister, Marie, who had already offered to help June by giving her eggs. Marie was taking the Pill and didn't think she would ever want children herself. June went with Marie to the clinic appointment to find out exactly what was involved; she didn't want her sister to run any risks. All three of them talked to the counsellor.

Marie came off the Pill and started fertility drugs, her treatment went smoothly and six eggs were collected and donated. They were fertilized with Ed's sperm and 3 days later June and Ed went back for the embryo transfer. June became pregnant, and when she went into labour Ed telephoned Marie, who rushed to the hospital and was the first to congratulate them.

19

Surrogacy

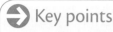
This chapter is very detailed and needs to be so if you are seriously considering surrogacy as an option. This chapter covers all you need to know if you are considering surrogacy for having children, or if you are considering being a surrogate mother.

Introduction

A surrogacy arrangement is when a woman, the surrogate mother, agrees to bear a child for another woman or couple, the intended parents, and give up the child at birth. The intended parents can adopt or take out a 'parental order' to become the legal parents of the child.

Surrogacy is a last resort where it is impossible or medically dangerous for the intended mother to carry the pregnancy herself.

Table 19.1 Surrogacy can be partial or full

Partial surrogacy (traditional or straight surrogacy)	Surrogate mother provides her egg as well as carrying the pregnancy. Sperm from the intended father is inseminated into the surrogate or IVF may be used
Full surrogacy	Surrogate mother makes no genetic contribution to the embryo. The egg is from the intended mother or a donor and the sperm from the intended father. The egg fertilizes in the test-tube and is placed into the surrogate's uterus to carry the pregnancy.

Some couples are infertile because the woman does not have a uterus (womb), either because she was born without one, or because it has been removed surgically for medical reasons (e.g. cancer, severe haemorrhage (bleeding), or rupture of the uterus during childbirth). Some women have had repeated miscarriage or have tried IVF many times without success and have given up hope of carrying their own pregnancy. Some women are medically advised not to undertake pregnancy because of dangerously high blood pressure, a heart condition, or liver disease.

Selection criteria

Couples wishing to be considered for IVF surrogacy will be asked for a referral letter from their GP giving the reasons for their surrogacy request and the background medical details.

The 'intended parents' (the couple requesting surrogacy) are seen for initial consultation (see Chapter 6). There is a lot to take in so you will also be given written information to take away and read later. The woman will be examined and the man is asked to provide a semen sample. If IVF surrogacy is suitable, the intended parents will be asked to bring the surrogate they have selected for an initial medical consultation at a later date.

Welfare of the child

The Human Fertilisation and Embryology Act (1990) requires that the welfare of the child must be taken into account before any treatment can commence at a licensed centre. This includes the welfare of any child born as a result of the treatment, and of any other existing children who may be affected by that birth. Many factors need to be taken into consideration in this assessment, including who would be legally responsible for any child born as a result of treatment, and who intends to bring up the child (see Chapter 5)

The doctor responsible for supervising the fertility treatment is responsible for making the final decision about whether or not treatment will be offered. Some fertility clinics refer surrogacy cases to the local Ethics Committee to make these clinical decisions. Names are omitted to protect confidentiality. If treatment is refused for any reason, the fertility clinic should explain the reasons and you can ask whether anything would persuade the fertility clinic to change its decision. Any remaining options should be explained and information about where to get counselling should be given.

Surrogacy and the law

Surrogacy is legal in the UK, but not in every country. British law states that any clinic providing treatment involving the donation of eggs and sperm, or the creation of embryos outside the body, must be licensed by the Human Fertilisation and Embryology Authority (HFEA). Therefore full surrogacy, which involves the creation of embryos outside the body, must only be performed in a licensed clinic. It is illegal for an individual or agency to act on a commercial (i.e. profit-making) basis to organize or assist a surrogacy arrangement for another person. Agencies or individuals may do this on a non-commercial basis and individual surrogate mothers may be paid expenses by the intended parents. Advertising that a person is willing to be a surrogate mother or that someone is looking for a surrogate mother is not allowed.

Are surrogacy arrangements enforceable by law?

Surrogacy arrangements are not enforceable by law. Therefore, whether or not a contract has been signed, and whether or not money has exchanged hands, either intended parents or surrogate could change their mind at any time. For this reason, it is particularly important that all parties have considered their decisions very carefully before going ahead with a surrogacy arrangement. If any of the parties have doubts about their commitment, they should say so before a pregnancy is established and the arrangement should not go ahead.

What is the legal status of the child?

UK law only recognizes the birth mother, i.e. the surrogate mother, as the legal mother. The legal father is more complicated. If the surrogate mother has a partner, he will be the legal father of the child, unless he can show that he did not consent to the treatment. If the surrogate mother does not have a partner and the treatment did not take place at a licensed clinic, i.e. it was self-insemination, the intended father will be the legal father. If treatment was undertaken in a licensed clinic and the surrogate has no partner, the child will be legally fatherless.

In order for the intended parents to become the legal parents of the child, they must either apply to adopt the child or apply for a parental order. This is true even if they are the genetic parents of the child (i.e. their sperm and eggs were used). If the intended parents change their minds about taking the child, for example if their circumstances have changed or if the child is born physically or mentally disabled and they feel unable to cope, the surrogate mother and her partner, if she has one, will be legally responsible for the child.

What is a parental order?

A parental order, which is obtainable by application to the courts, makes the intended parents, become the child's legal parents. This has the same effect as adoption, but allows a quicker route in cases of surrogacy. See information on parental orders on p. 147–148.

A child born to a surrogate mother will be registered as her child and that of the legal father. Where a parental order has been granted a separate entry will be made in the Parental Orders Register. It is not possible to abolish the original birth certificate, and at the age of 18 the child will be able to obtain a certified copy of the original record which will include the name of the surrogate mother. Prior to being given access to this information the person will be advised that counselling is available.

Take legal advice from a solicitor

It is advisable that all parties (intended parents and surrogate) take independent legal advice from a solicitor who practises in family law. The following points should be considered.

◆ The procedures necessary to change the legal parentage for a parental order: the solicitor will need a report from the counsellor that counselling took place to put before the court.

◆ The need to take out insurance cover for the surrogate mother and her family in the event of complications during pregnancy and birth, and for a reasonable interval after birth.

◆ The need to make appropriate wills. All parties should make appropriate arrangements for the future of the child in the event of accident or death. The intended parents should also appoint guardians.

What are reasonable expenses?

You will want to decide between you what you feel are reasonable expenses, but it is not unusual for payments to total £10 000. Careful records of expenses paid to the host and, where appropriate, receipts should be kept. Loss of earnings as a result of pregnancy would be allowable but claiming loss of earnings where no earnings existed might jeopardize the change in parentage. Unforeseen delays and complications in pregnancy might increase the expenses.

'Unreasonable expenses' would be against the law. The courts may authorize payments; in one case the court made a retrospective authorization.

Who is suitable to be a surrogate mother?

A potential surrogate mother must be in good overall health and be able to undergo a pregnancy with the minimum risk to her own health. Some medical conditions will prevent a woman becoming a surrogate mother, for example if there are any known medical conditions that could lead to complications in the pregnancy or put the woman at risk. Those who are considerably overweight, heavy smokers or drinkers, or substance abusers are not suitable as surrogate mothers because of the risks to both the woman and the baby.

A potential surrogate mother should have had at least one child of her own

As the risks of illness and problems are much higher in the first pregnancy, it is strongly recommended that a surrogate mother should have borne at least one child previously and preferably have completed her own family. This also means that the woman is able to give informed consent to the arrangement, because she already knows what pregnancy and childbirth is like. Only in very exceptional circumstances should a woman who has not had a child herself consider becoming a surrogate mother.

A potential surrogate mother should be less than 35 years old

Because of the increased risks of Down syndrome resulting from the eggs of an older woman, an upper age limit is set for those donating eggs to other women. Therefore the age limit should also apply to surrogate mothers whose own eggs are to be used, and because the risks of pregnancy increase with age, any woman over 35 should give careful consideration before deciding to become a surrogate mother.

A potential surrogate mother should have the support of her partner and family

Being a surrogate mother is emotionally and physically demanding.

It is important that a woman thinking about being a surrogate has the backing of her partner, family, or friends to provide emotional support and practical help during and after the pregnancy. Surrogacy is not something to enter into lightly. Careful thought must be given to the medical, emotional, legal, and practical issues, and to the implications of parting with the child at birth. Thought must also be given to the effect on any existing children and on the potential surrogate's partner, family, and friends.

A surrogate mother should have the support of her partner and family.

What is the level of medical involvement?

The amount of medical assistance required will depend upon the individual circumstances. There will be considerable medical involvement at the beginning with IVF treatment, which will be carried out in a fertility clinic. If you are thinking about surrogacy speak to your GP who can provide advice and support and will want to know the medical details that may be relevant in looking after you.

The importance of screening tests

In surrogacy arrangements there is a risk that infections such as HIV or hepatitis could be passed to the surrogate mother from the intended parents, through the sperm or eggs. For this reason it is strongly recommended that those involved have testing to minimize the risk. Where treatment is given in a licensed clinic, the intended father and the intended mother, if her eggs are to be used, are tested for HIV, hepatitis, and other infectious diseases. Usually the sperm and the embryos are stored, in quarantine, whilst repeat tests are carried out to minimize the risk of passing on any infection. The surrogate mother will also be tested for her blood group and antibodies and to ensure that she has no infection. Before having the tests, you should think about what it would mean if the result were positive.

The benefits of counselling

Although offering to become a surrogate mother for an infertile couple might appear to be an uncomplicated altruistic act, it is not an easy course of action. Equally, whilst the intended parents may see surrogacy as the answer to their prayers, they are also likely to have worries about the planned course of action.

All parties must be clear about the implications of their actions before going ahead.

A potential surrogate mother must think carefully about how she might feel about the developing child, the possibility of miscarriage or termination, and the effect of parting with the child if the pregnancy is successful. The intended mother may worry about her potential ability to bond with a child carried by another woman or fear that the surrogate mother will decide to keep the child. Both the surrogate mother and the intended parents will need to consider carefully how they would react if the child was born physically or mentally disabled, what they would wish to do, and how this would affect their surrogacy arrangement. All these issues should be aired in counselling. While appropriate counselling cannot eradicate all the worries that go with fertility treatments generally and surrogacy in particular, specially trained and knowledgeable counsellors can provide reassurance that the varied emotions experienced by people in this situation are not unusual.

Counselling is offered to those taking part in a surrogacy arrangement. Those making their own arrangements should also see a counsellor to help think through the issues and the implications of the arrangement. Most general practitioners will be able to provide details of the counselling services available in the area, or a list of counsellors can be obtained from the British Infertility Counselling Association (see 'Useful addresses').

Health risks to the surrogate mother

The risk of transmitting infection, such as HIV or hepatitis, to the surrogate mother from the intended parents has been discussed in the section on the importance of screening. Testing can reduce the risk, and if the embryos are quarantined, the risk is very small.

In full surrogacy, when more than one embryo is placed in the surrogate mother's uterus (womb), the risk of multiple pregnancy increases. Around 20–25 per cent of the pregnancies resulting from IVF will result in a multiple pregnancy of twins or triplets, depending on the number of embryos replaced. This carries risks for both mothers and babies, and there are serious implications for the intended parents in raising children from a multiple pregnancy. In view of this high risk of multiple pregnancy, it is normal for no more than two embryos to be replaced.

Surrogacy pregnancies have the same effect on a woman's physical health as any other pregnancy (apart from the risks associated with multiple pregnancy). The surrogate mother should be aware of the usual risks of pregnancy before going ahead. In very rare cases pregnancy can result in maternal death (six deaths per 100 000 pregnancies per year), but less serious problems, such as pregnancy diabetes, high blood pressure, urinary tract infections, haemorrhage, stress urinary incontinence, painful intercourse, and haemorrhoids, are more common. The intended parents should buy insurance cover for the surrogate mother and her family in the event of any misfortune.

There is also a risk that the surrogate mother may suffer from postnatal depression. This can occur after any pregnancy, but the surrogate mother may also feel a great sense of loss and bereavement at being separated from the baby she has carried for 9 months.

Are there any health risks to the baby?

Some couples are infertile because the woman was born without a uterus (womb). This is called Meyer–Rokitansky–Kuster–Hauser syndrome. The evidence suggests that this syndrome is not inherited and that any children born are unlikely to have the same problem.

Once an arrangement has been made, and before pregnancy, a number of decisions need to be made about the pregnancy.

Decisions to be made about the pregnancy

Tests during the pregnancy

You will need to decide whether to have tests such as ultrasound or blood tests, amniocentesis, or chorionic villus sampling (CVS) to detect chromosome abnormalities. Thought must also be given, in advance, about what to do if a severe abnormality is detected. For example, if the intended parents feel that they would be unable to look after a child with a severe disability and the surrogate mother is opposed to termination, the parties need to decide how the situation should be managed and if agreement cannot be reached, the surrogacy arrangement should not go ahead. When it happens, a party may change their mind, but discussing the matter in advance should minimize this happening.

Ideally, a joint decision should be reached between the surrogate mother and the intended parents, although there may be times when their views differ. It is important that the issues are discussed before the surrogacy arrangement proceeds.

> It should be clear to everyone involved that the surrogate mother, with the advice of health professionals where appropriate, will make the final decision during and immediately after the pregnancy.

The preferred method of delivery

It is important to know, for example, if the surrogate mother wishes to give birth in water or if the intended parents are totally opposed to the use of drugs in labour. Again discussion should take place before the pregnancy. The surrogate mother, with the advice of health professionals, should make final decisions. Other decisions need to be taken immediately after the delivery about which parents would normally be consulted, such as in the case of a premature birth. Ideally, a joint decision should be reached, but the surrogate mother has the right to make decisions about the child immediately after delivery. In the days after delivery, provided that the child has been passed to the intended parents, responsibilities for decision-making pass to them.

Will the surrogate mother have contact with the intended parents and the child?

This depends on the individual circumstances and the wishes of the parties concerned. It is important that this is discussed from the beginning, so that problems do not develop at a later stage. Some surrogate mothers find it helpful to have the support of the intended parents throughout the pregnancy, and the intended parents often want to share the experience and be involved with the pregnancy, such as attending hospital for scans and possibly being present at, or immediately after, the birth. Others prefer to have limited contact.

Once the child is born, the level of contact will again depend on the wishes of the individuals concerned. In some cases, all agree that contact should stop as soon as the child is handed to the intended parents, except for the communication required for transferring legal parentage of the child. In other cases the intended parents will send photographs of the child to the surrogate mother, and in some cases the child will know the surrogate mother and her own family.

> What is important is that the surrogate mother and intended parents agree on what level of contact is best for them.

Who else might be affected by the surrogacy arrangement?

The main parties are the intended parents and the surrogate mother, but the effect on other family members, such as the surrogate mother's partner, her parents, and any existing children, needs to be considered.

Partner

The partner may feel a sense of bereavement at losing the child his partner has carried for the previous 9 months.

Brothers and sisters

Unless sensitively handled, existing children may be disturbed by the loss of a sibling and fear that they may also be 'given away'.

Intended parents' family

The child's grandparents may find it difficult to accept the method of the child's conception and may treat him/her differently from other grandchildren. Other children may find it difficult to accept their new brother and sister and may resent the attention given to the child from the parents. With careful handling, all these difficulties can be faced, but need some thought before deciding to go ahead.

What are the implications for the child?

One question that all intended parents have to deal with, is whether to tell the child about his/her origins.

> Research shows that most people who have children conceived from surrogacy decide to explain the conception and birth to the child.

If parents decide not to tell, they face a number of difficulties. Surrogacy is difficult to conceal from others, and if other people know about the arrangement, there is the chance that the child may find out. The experience of learning in this way and the discovery of deception by his/her parents may be very distressing for a child. Another factor to be considered is that at the age of 18 the child will have the legal right to discover the identity of his/her surrogate mother.

The number of children born as a result of surrogacy arrangements is small, and there is a very limited research available into the effects on the child. However, it has been suggested that such children may feel a certain amount of anxiety about being 'different' from their friends and may sometimes feel pressure to live up to the expectations of their parents, who went to such great lengths to have them. However, these concerns do not seem to reflect the reality for children from other 'different' families, such as those resulting from infertility treatment or adoption.

> Positively, it has been suggested that children conceived via surrogacy arrangements may in fact be proud of their parents' courage and grateful to their parents, and the surrogate mother, for their existence.

IVF treatment

Treatment of the intended parents requires stimulation of the ovaries, as in normal IVF (see Chapter 14), with monitoring of the cycle, collection of the eggs by vaginal ultrasound-guided needle aspiration, insemination of the eggs, and freezing of any resulting embryos. The embryos are then kept frozen for 6 months. HIV (AIDS) testing is repeated at the end of this time, and when all the tests have proved negative arrangements are made for the surrogate to receive the embryos.

Embryos may be transferred to the surrogate in a hormone-controlled cycle which requires taking a drug to stop the host's own menstrual cycle, followed by a course of oestrogen tablets to build up the lining of the womb and later by progesterone injections. Alternatively, if cycles are perfectly regular and if there is no chance of pregnancy occurring, a natural cycle transfer will be considered.

The chance of pregnancy occurring in any one treatment cycle is in the region of 20–30 per cent. Normally only two embryos are transferred in order to reduce the chance of multiple pregnancy.

Pregnancy testing is arranged 16 days after the transfer. If this is positive an ultrasound scan is arranged. Once pregnancy is confirmed, surrogate mothers are referred to their GP to arrange obstetric care. The GP and other health workers will need to know that this is a surrogacy case so that the care can be properly arranged.

Consent to the storage and use of gametes

In all cases, people giving consent to the storage and/or use of their gametes (eggs or sperm) or embryos produced from them may change or withdraw their consent at any time up until the genetic material has been introduced into the surrogate, i.e. the embryos have been replaced.

HFEA register

The HFEA keeps a confidential register of information about donors, patients, and treatments (see Chapter 17).

Registration of birth in surrogacy cases

The surrogate parents (birth mother and her partner/husband) are the legal parents of a child born through a surrogacy arrangement until legal parentage is transferred to the commissioning couple. Therefore the surrogate mother must register the baby to whom she has given birth in the normal way. Her husband or partner should normally be registered as the partner.

When a parental order has been granted by the court the Registrar General will make an entry in a separate Parental Order Register re-registering the child. This will be cross-referenced with the entry in the Register of Births. It will not be possible for the public to make a link between entries in the Register of Births and the Parental Order Register. It will be possible for adults who are the subject of parental orders to gain access, after being offered counselling, to their original birth certificates.

What happens now?

Surrogacy might be the only opportunity for some people to have children, but it is not something to enter into lightly. It is a good idea to obtain as much information as possible, take time to reflect on it, and if possible discuss it with partner, family, or friends. Anyone with doubts about their commitment should not go ahead.

 Personal history

Roopa and Mohammed were planning a family. As a child, Roopa had an operation for a cancer on her ovary. This required major life-saving surgery followed by chemotherapy. Roopa was having periods and had been told that the fertility outlook was good. When the details of treatment were obtained, it showed that part of the uterus and one ovary had been removed. MRI scan showed one remaining ovary and just the cervix. Surrogacy using eggs from her ovary was the only option.

Application for a parental order

In order to apply for a parental order, the following criteria must be met.

◆ The child must be genetically related to one or both of the intended parents.

◆ The intended parents must be married to each other and must both be aged 18 or over.

◆ The legal mother and father (i.e. surrogate mother and her partner, if she has one) must consent to the making of the order (this consent cannot be given until 6 weeks after the birth of the child).

- No money other than reasonable expenses has been paid for the surrogacy arrangement unless the payment has been authorized by a court.

- The child must be living with the intended parents and one or both of the intended must be living in the UK.

- An application must be made within 6 months of the birth of the child.

Parental orders in surrogacy cases

The following conditions must be fulfilled before a parental order can be granted.

- The child must be genetically related to at least one of the commissioning couple.

- The surrogate parents must have consented to making the order (unless they are incapable of giving consent or are untraceable) no earlier than 6 weeks after the birth of the child.

- The intended parents must be married to each other, and both must be aged 18 or over.

- The intended parents must have applied for an order within 6 months of the child's birth

- No money, other than expenses, must have been paid in respect of the surrogacy arrangement, unless authorized by a court.

- The child must be living with the intended parents.

- The intended parents must be living in the UK, the Channel Islands, or the Isle of Man.

Application forms for parental orders are available from Family Proceedings Courts (Magistrates Courts) in the intended parents' home area. Legal aid may be available to cover parental order proceedings.

20

Fertility and the older woman

> ## ➜ Key points
>
> ◆ Couples are increasingly choosing to have children later. The number of new mothers over the age of 40 in the UK has increased by 50 per cent over the last 10 years.
>
> ◆ Fertility in women, as well as the success rate from fertility treatment, decreases significantly from age 35.
>
> ◆ The chances of miscarriage increase with age from one in every six pregnancies to one in every three pregnancies by age 40.
>
> ◆ The chances of a woman giving birth to a baby with Down syndrome also increase with age: one in 200 women at age 38, one in 100 at age 40, and one in 30 at age 45.

Egg numbers, fertility, and menopause

Women's fertility is very dependent on age. Girls are born with all the eggs for their lifetime already present in the ovaries. In fact, the number of eggs is greatest before birth at over a million, and there is a steady loss of eggs even before the onset of monthly periods in the teens. During adult life, several eggs start to develop each month, but usually only one egg matures and is released at ovulation and the others die. Egg numbers are estimated at around 25 000 at age 37. The process of egg loss becomes faster in the late thirties and forties, and less than 1000 eggs are left by the age of 50.

Menopause means the last menstrual period, and the average age is 51 for women in the UK. Some women will have the menopause later than this, but others will experience an early menopause, and for one woman in 100 this happens before the age of 40. Smoking is known to cause an earlier menopause. Treatment for cancer using chemotherapy also causes early menopause by destroying some of the store of eggs. A tendency towards early menopause can also run in families.

Pregnancy rates

Fertility falls from the mid-thirties, and this affects success rates from fertility treatment as well as natural pregnancy. Couples trying for pregnancy when the woman is under 30 have an 85 per cent (85 out of 100) chance of conceiving within a year. This falls to 75 per cent at 30, 66 per cent at 35, and 44 per cent at 40.

For many women, fertility ceases 8–10 years before the menopause. This has been studied in societies which do not use contraception for religious or cultural reasons. Often these couples have large families but typically the last child is born when the woman is 42. There is a slight trend towards later menopause (and thus prolonged fertility) in modern societies where women are healthier than ever before. Several celebrities have become parents relatively late: Madonna had a baby at 41 and Cherie Blair at 45 whilst her husband was Prime Minister. However, only a minority of women will be able to conceive at this age.

Fertility tests and treatment

It is important to be referred for fertility help quickly if you are older. Ask your GP for referral if you are aged over 35 and have been trying to conceive for more than 6 months. There may be nothing wrong, but if you have a fertility problem it needs to be addressed promptly. Success rates for treatment fall as a woman gets older; for example IVF birth rates are 10 per cent at best for women over the age of 40 (only 10 in 100 will conceive and give birth) and there have been no births from IVF in the UK to women over 45 (unless donor eggs are used).

Many women in their late thirties and forties will be ovulating regularly, but they may not be able to conceive if their eggs are not of good quality. It is difficult to assess this, as it is not possible to examine eggs directly (except in IVF). In contrast, sperm quality can be examined easily by studying a semen sample under the microscope. Therefore indirect tests of ovarian function are used for women. These can include a timed blood test for hormone measurements in the first few days of the menstrual cycle, and an ultrasound scan to count small follicles (see Chapter 7 and Figure 7.3).

During fertility treatment such as IVF, the body's response to fertility drugs will also give an idea of ovarian function and egg quality; usually the more eggs the better the chance of pregnancy!

Miscarriage and Down syndrome

The chance of having a miscarriage rises with age, from a background rate of one in six pregnancies to a risk of one in three by age 40. This increase in the risk of miscarriage is believed to be caused by abnormalities in the egg or early embryo which prevent it from developing.

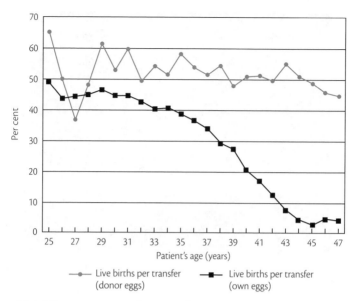

Figure 20.1 IVF pregnancy rates using women's own eggs and donor eggs (2003 data from Centers for Disease Control and Prevention, USA).

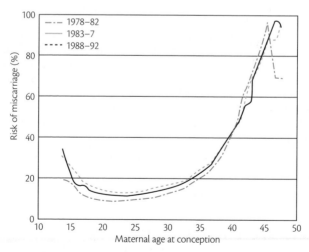

Figure 20.2 The risk of miscarriage at different ages. Nybo Anderson *et al.* Maternal age and fetal loss: population based register linkage study, *British Medical Journal*, **320**:1708–12, (2000), with permission from the BMJ Publishing Group.

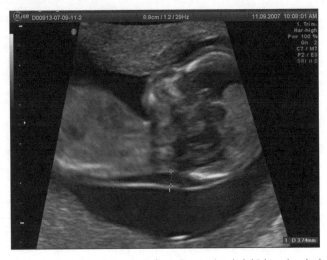

Figure 20.3 Ultrasound scan of 12-week fetus showing 'nuchal thickness' at the back of the neck (marked with crosses).

There is also a higher chance of chromosome abnormalities in the egg, giving rise to the birth of a baby with Down syndrome. This affects one in 200 women at the age of 38, rising to one in 100 at 40, and at least one in 30 at 45. Special tests for chromosome abnormalities, including Down syndrome, will be offered in the antenatal clinic from 12 weeks of pregnancy. In the first instance, you may be offered an ultrasound scan to check the 'nuchal thickness' (a measurement on the back of the baby's neck), perhaps combined with a blood test for pregnancy hormones; together these can give an estimate of the likelihood of your baby having Down syndrome. If you are at high risk and want to have a definite answer, you will be offered amniocentesis which takes a sample of fluid from the womb at around 16 weeks of pregnancy. Unfortunately this carries a risk of miscarriage of up to one in 100. CVS (chorionic villus sampling) can be done earlier but takes a sample from the placenta and carries a higher risk of losing the pregnancy.

Preimplantation screening (PGS) can be used to try to avoid these problems (see below and Chapter 16).

In egg donation pregnancies, the risk of miscarriage and Down syndrome is related to the age of the egg donor.

Aneuploidy screening

Aneuploidy screening, which is also called preimplantation genetic screening (PGS), is a new technique of embryo screening. It is increasingly used by older women going through IVF, so that embryos can be screened for Down syndrome and similar conditions before they are replaced in the womb. This should improve the success rate of treatment and reduce the risk of miscarriage, but it is not yet proven. We still need more information on the safety and effectiveness of PGS (see Chapter 16).

Pregnancy in older mothers

Couples are choosing to have children later, and in the UK there are now more women giving birth in their thirties than their twenties. The number of new mothers over 40 has increased by 50 per cent over the last 10 years and includes many women who have suffered from years of infertility. The outlook is good for both mothers and babies, but pregnancy complications are more common when women are older.

High blood pressure and pre-eclampsia are more common in older mothers, and so is pregnancy diabetes. These conditions tend to occur in the second half of pregnancy. They need close monitoring and may lead to early delivery. Twin pregnancy greatly increases these risks.

Labour and birth tend to be faster and easier in younger women, especially those who have given birth before. Medical help is more likely to be needed by first-time mothers and older mothers. Up to half of women having their first child over the age of 40 will deliver by Caesarean section. For parents and staff, the most important thing is the safe delivery of a healthy child.

The risks of pregnancy increase in women over 50, and this is one of the reasons why most fertility clinics in the UK do not offer egg donation treatment over this age. The oldest woman to give birth in the UK was 63 when she had a son by Caesarean section in 2006.

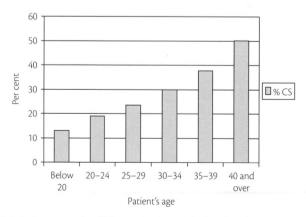

Figure 20.4 Caesarean section (CS) rates for women having their first baby at different ages (Canadian data from K. S. Joseph *et al.*, *Obstet Gynecol* **105**:1410–18, 2005).

Case study

Rebecca was 38 when she had a miscarriage. She and Paul had been together for nearly 10 years but had busy careers and had only tried for children after getting married 2 years previously. Rebecca felt devastated by the miscarriage and for several months she couldn't bear to think about trying again.

When they did try again, nothing happened. It was a year before they went to get advice because Rebecca's periods had become irregular. Their consultant said that her ovaries were not working well even for a 40-year-old and her eggs were poor quality.

They decided to try IVF, but the treatment had to be cancelled because Rebecca did not respond to the drugs, and she was told that she could not become pregnant with her own eggs. This was the worst news yet, but strangely they felt more determined to go on in their quest for a family. They contacted an adoption agency, and also went back to the IVF clinic to discuss egg donation. Because of the shortage of donors in the UK, they are now planning to have treatment in the USA where Paul's family live.

21

Gynaecological problems and fertility

> **➲ Key points**
>
> ◆ Gynaecological problems can cause infertility and coexist with infertility.
>
> ◆ Moderate and severe endometriosis results in adhesions (scarring) and is linked with fertility problems, whereas women with minimal to mild endometriosis have no significant decrease in the chance of getting pregnant.
>
> ◆ Fibroids can sometimes cause infertility as well as problems during pregnancy.
>
> ◆ Most ovarian cysts are part of the monthly ovarian cycle and don't require treatment. If they persist, they may be aspirated for cytological examination or removed surgically.

Infertility can be caused by gynaecological problems, and gynaecological problems can coexist with infertility. In this chapter we discuss some of the common gynaecological problems and their treatment.

Endometriosis

Endometriosis is commonly found at laparoscopy in women who have had children as well as in women who are infertile. It is not a cancer and rarely changes into a cancer. It can cause pain: painful periods, pain for several days before a period, and pain on intercourse. It can also be found without symptoms.

Endometriosis is graded into minimal to mild, moderate, and severe depending on how much of the pelvis is affected. The more severe the disease, the smaller the chance of getting pregnant naturally. Women with minimal to mild endometriosis have almost the same chance of getting pregnant as women with a 'perfect pelvis'. Moderate and severe endometriosis result in adhesions and are linked with fertility problems.

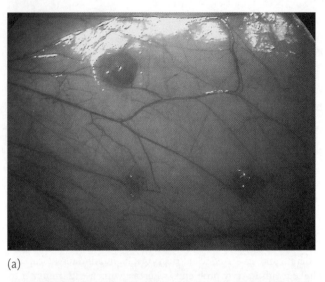

(a)

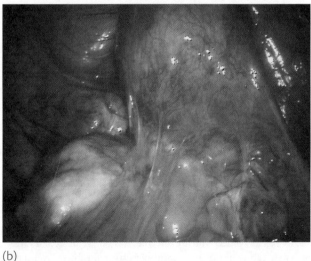

(b)

Figure 21.1 (a) Mild endometriosis, showing spots of endometriosis on the skin lining the abdomen, seen at laparoscopy. (b) Severe endometriosis; it is no longer possible to see the tubes or ovaries clearly.

Medical or drug treatment for endometriosis has never been shown to improve pregnancy rates. Treatment is effective for pain linked with endometriosis and is also used in preparation for further surgery.

Surgical treatment of endometriosis

The aim of surgical treatment is to destroy or cut out (excise) nodules of endometriosis and release adhesions around the ovaries or Fallopian tubes.

Endometriosis can cause ovarian cysts, which are removed surgically (ovarian cystectomy) in women trying to get pregnant. It is reasonable to leave small endometriotic cysts, but cysts larger than 4 centimetres in diameter are generally removed. This involves shelling out the cyst from inside the ovary. If the cyst is simply drained, it re-forms. Surgical removal of the cyst improves the chance of getting pregnant naturally and improves access to the ovaries if IVF is considered (see Chapter 14).

Surgical treatment of minimal to mild endometriosis improves the chance of getting pregnant. In a study which compared pregnancy rates after surgical treatment and laparoscopy alone, pregnancy rates were higher after surgical treatment. This was a good study and answered an important question about whether surgical treatment of endometriosis helped women conceive, but it was criticized because some women were told that they had had treatment before they went home. Some women had surgical treatment for endometriosis as well as release of adhesions that could have affected the results. After surgical treatment, it would be reasonable to wait a year to see if pregnancy happens naturally, unless there are other fertility factors such as maternal age or male factor infertility.

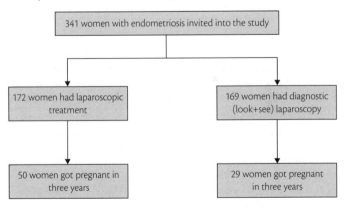

Figure 21.2 Laparoscopic (keyhole) surgery to treat endometriosis improves pregnancy rates.

When a woman is in pain, surgery is the best treatment for moderate and severe endometriosis. Surgical treatment improves pregnancy rates and helps to relieve pain. IVF is an alternative to surgery or can be offered following surgery if pregnancy doesn't happen naturally. Drawbacks of surgery include post-operative adhesion formation and incomplete removal of the disease with return of pain.

What treatment to choose will depend on the severity of endometriosis, your age, how long you have been trying to get pregnant, whether you have ever been pregnant, and the presence of other fertility factors such as blocked tubes or male factor infertility.

Fertility treatment and endometriosis

The best treatment for women with minimal to mild endometriosis who are trying to get pregnant is to boost fertility by combining ovarian stimulation and intrauterine insemination. One in six women will get pregnant per cycle of treatment and most of the pregnancies (80 per cent) happen in the first few cycles of treatment. If a couple are not pregnant after three or four cycles, it is usual to advise IVF. If too many follicles develop, treatment can either be stopped or converted to IVF.

Ovarian stimulation and intra-uterine insemination

For successful treatment:

- women should be under the age of 38
- the Fallopian tubes should be healthy
- periods (ovulation) should be regular
- endometriosis should be minimal or mild
- there should be no severe male factor fertility problem.

In vitro fertilization

IVF and embryo transfer is an established and successful treatment for endometriosis-related infertility. IVF is suitable for women with damaged or blocked tubes, moderate or severe endometriosis, and minimal to mild endometriosis with male factor fertility problems, and for women who have failed to conceive by intra-uterine insemination.

The use of a gonadotrophin-releasing hormone (GnRH) agonist results in high pregnancy and live birth rates. This is because fewer cycles are cancelled and a premature hormone surge is prevented. Other advantages include more eggs for collection (and more embryos) and the ability to time the treatment and egg collection. Several GnRH agonist protocols for ovarian stimulation are available, and each has advantages and disadvantages.

- Treating a woman with moderate–severe endometriosis with GnRH agonist before IVF improves pregnancy rates.
- Treatment with GnRH agonist for 2–7 months before IVF resulted in higher pregnancy rates than those in women treated for the standard 7 days.

In the past, women with moderate to severe endometriosis have been shown to have lower pregnancy rates than women with minimal to mild endometriosis. However, treatment with GnRH agonists after surgical treatment results in good pregnancy rates comparable with other causes of infertility. The presence of small endometriosis cysts on the ovaries does not reduce the success of IVF treatment, but there is an increased risk of developing a pelvic infection following transvaginal oocyte collection. This is because the old blood within the cyst may leak into the pelvis during egg collection.

Fibroids

Fibroids are common in women who have had children and women who are trying to get pregnant. It is not always necessary to remove a fibroid if it is discovered during fertility tests, as fibroids do not always cause infertility.

Fibroids are made up of fibrous tissue within the muscle of the womb. They are not a cancer and only rarely develop into cancer. When they do, they enlarge rapidly.

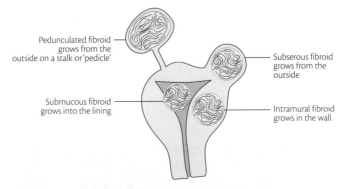

Pedunculated fibroid grows from the outside on a stalk or 'pedicle'

Subserous fibroid grows from the outside

Submucous fibroid grows into the lining

Intramural fibroid grows in the wall

Figure 21.3 Fibroids are named depending on where in the uterus they are growing.

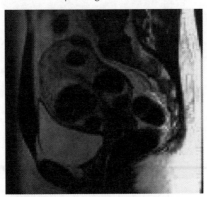

Figure 21.4 MRI picture of different types of fibroids.

Fibroids can be found within the muscle of the womb, sticking out from the surface (subserous fibroid), within the wall of the womb (intramural fibroid), or sticking into the lining of the womb (submucous fibroid).

Fibroids and pregnancy

Fibroids can sometimes cause problems during pregnancy. They grow during pregnancy and can soften, undergoing a change called red degeneration which causes pain. Pregnant women with fibroids have an increased chance of bleeding, premature labour, breech presentation, Caesarean delivery, retained placenta, and bleeding after the delivery (postpartum haemorrhage).

Submucous fibroids are commonly linked with fertility problems. They are thought to act as a 'coil' interfering with implantation of the embryo within the lining of the womb. Your gynaecologist will suggest removal of this type of fibroid by an operation called transcervical resection of fibroid.

Transcervical resection of fibroid

A small telescope is passed through the cervix and the fibroid is 'shaved away' using a heated wire. The fibroid is removed in pieces (called chips) through the cervix. The operation is normally carried out under general anaesthetic as a day case. Your gynaecologist may suggest a pre-operative course of treatment to shrink the fibroid and reduce its blood supply before surgery.

There is debate about when and how the other types of fibroids should removed. In general, fibroids larger than 5 centimetres in diameter are removed because

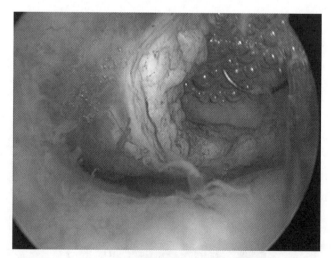

Figure 21.5 Transcervical resection of fibroid. The fibroid is shaved away inside the lining of the womb.

they may be linked with fertility and can enlarge during, pregnancy causing pain or pregnancy problems.

Myomectomy

In general, fertility tests should be completed to ensure that there are no other fertility problems before embarking on surgery.

Myomectomy may be performed laparoscopically or through a bigger cut on the tummy. In a comparison of the two types of surgery, there was no difference in pregnancy rates afterwards. The operation is normally carried out under general anaesthetic. You will need to stay in hospital for a few days until you are well enough to go home. Your gynaecologist may suggest a preoperative course of treatment to shrink the fibroid and reduce its blood supply before surgery.

Surgery leaves a scar, both on the skin and also on the uterus (womb). It can also result in scar tissue within the pelvis, called adhesions. These adhesions are similar to cobwebs and bind structures together. They can reduce fertility by trapping the tube or getting in the way so that the egg cannot be picked up from the ovary. The number of adhesions that form will depend on the skill of your surgeon and your own healing.

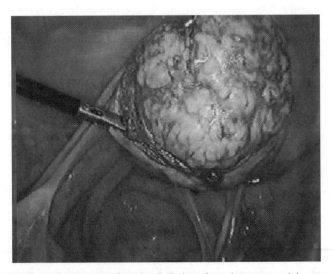

Figure 21.6 Myomectomy. The fibroid is shelled out from the uterus and the uterus is stitched back up.

In order to minimize the chance of adhesion formation, your surgeon will try to:

◆ make as few cuts on the womb as possible (fewer cuts = less scar tissue formation)

◆ reduce bleeding to a minimum by injecting a hormone to shrink the blood vessels at the time of the surgery, as well as pre-operative treatment to reduce the size of the fibroid and its blood supply.

The fibroid is shelled out from the muscle and bleeding is to be expected. You may be anaemic after the operation and even need a blood transfusion. Before the operation you should aim to build up your iron stores by eating a balanced diet rich in iron and taking an iron supplement. On rare occasions (fewer than one in 200 operations) hysterectomy has to be carried out because the bleeding is uncontrollable. This is only done in a life-saving situation, when the woman has already lost a lot of blood and there is still uncontrolled bleeding.

After myomectomy, you may be advised to have a planned Caesarean section if the fibroid was large or the lining of the womb was entered. After most myomectomies, it is safe to try for normal delivery. This will depend on how many fibroids were removed and where from. Your surgeon will help you make this decision.

Alternatives to surgery for the treatment of fibroids

Medical treatment with anti-hormones

Alternative treatment is usually only temporary. Medical treatment with a GnRH agonist stops periods and shrinks the fibroid, but is contraceptive. Treatment can usually be given for 3–6 months, but maximum shrinkage is usually seen after 3 months. The fibroid usually grows rapidly after treatment is stopped, and returns to its previous size.

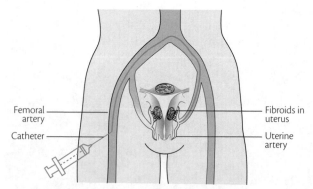

Figure 21.7 Uterine artery embolization. This treatment involves blocking the uterine artery with particles injected through the artery in the groins. Reproduced from Sadler *et al. Women's Health* (*Oxford General Practice Library*) (2007), with permission from Oxford University Press.

Uterine artery embolization

This treatment involves blocking the uterine arteries with particles injected via the femoral and uterine arteries. It is carried out under local anaesthetic and many women are in hospital for as little as 24–36 hours, with advice to rest for 1–2 weeks. Pain is normal after the procedure. The blood supply of the fibroid is reduced and the fibroid can shrink by up to half its size.

The most commonly reported complications are the need for hysterectomy in 0.5 per cent (2/400 women) to 11.8 per cent (6/51 women) and late expulsion of a fibroid in 2.2 per cent (9/400) to 7.7 per cent (2/26) of women. Other complications include infection and fever. One death was reported in a small study of 21 women.

The ovaries are very sensitive to radiation and there have been reports of premature menopause following the treatment. Premature menopause after uterine artery embolization is more common in women over 45 because of reduced ovarian reserve. Because the safety of this procedure is not fully established, it is recommended only to women whose fibroids are causing symptoms and who would otherwise need an operation.

In three studies totalling 604 women, 24 (4 per cent) reported pregnancies following uterine artery embolization. However, it was unclear how many women in these studies wished to get pregnant. No long-term data about its safety are available, and it has been suggested that babies born after uterine artery embolization are smaller. It is not recommended for women who are actively trying to get pregnant.

MRI-guided percutaneous laser ablation of uterine fibroids

This treatment involves injecting the fibroid directly and heating it from within. Needles are inserted after a local anaesthetic and the procedure is carried out under sedation. MRI is used to guide the placement of the needle. The fibroid shrinks as a result of the treatment. Again, there are no long-term data about its safety. The treatment is very specialized and currently only one centre in the UK undertakes it.

MRI-guided transcutaneous focused ultrasound ablation for uterine fibroids

High-intensity focused ultrasound has been used to destroy liver tumours and is the newest treatment for fibroids. MRI assists in directing the treatment. There are no long-term data on its safety or on fibroid recurrence. This treatment is only available in certain hospitals.

Abnormalities in the shape of the womb (uterine anomalies)

While inside our mother's tummies, the womb begins as two halves which join to become a single womb with one cervix (entrance to the womb). This process of fusion is complicated and abnormalities are common, being found in as many as one in 20 women.

The most common variation is the bicornuate or heart-shaped womb. This shape is not linked with fertility problems and does not require any treatment or surgery. It is thought to make breech birth more likely, but in practice breech remains rare.

Where the two halves have partially joined, there is a division or septum between the two halves. The septum is made up of fibrous tissue and has less blood supply. This is thought to affect the development of the normal pregnancy. This abnormality is linked with late miscarriage and premature birth, but there is debate about whether this is linked with fertility problems.

Treatment is always suggested if there is a past history of repeated late miscarriage. The septate uterus can be treated by operative hysteroscopy. The septum is cut with scissors, wire, or laser, with no obvious advantage of one type of operation over the other. A coil may be left to prevent adhesions forming between one wall and the other while healing takes place. Whether a septate uterus discovered incidentally during fertility tests requires treatment is not known.

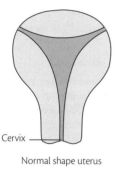

Cervix — Normal shape uterus

Cervix — Bicornuate or heart-shaped uterus

Figure 21.8 Uterine shape variations.

Ovarian cysts

It is common for ovarian cysts to be discovered during the course of an ultrasound scan. Most ovarian cysts are physiological; that is, they are part of the monthly ovarian cycle and require no treatment. They will simply disappear with time.

If the cyst persists after one or two periods, it may be aspirated transvaginally and fluid sent for cytology. If it re-forms, surgical removal is required.

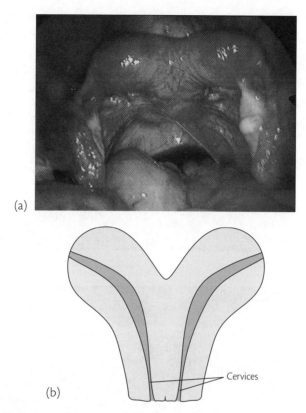

(a)

(b)

Cervices

Figure 21.9 Laparoscopic picture and diagram to show a double uterus. This woman will have two cervices (uterus didelphus).

> ❌ **Myth:** It is generally thought that a cyst sticks out from the ovary, like a bobble on the outside.
>
> ❗ **Fact:** The cyst is within the ovary. If you imagine the ovary as an orange, the segments inside are the cyst and the peel is the ovary. Alternatively, the ovary can be envisaged a hard-boiled egg and the cyst as the egg yolk. The ovary will still 'work' and produce an egg each month. Surgically removing an ovarian cyst involves cutting the ovary and shelling out the cyst. Like oranges, they can be easy or difficult to peel!

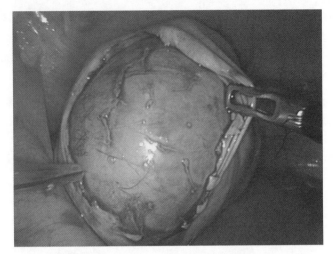

(a) Removal of cyst

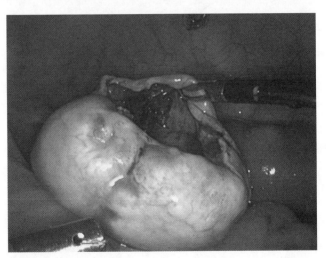

(b) Operation complete

Figure 21.10 Surgical removal of a cyst from within the ovary.

Endometrioma

An endometrioma or endometriotic cyst is a blood-filled cyst and has a typical appearance on scan. This is described as a ground-glass appearance. If it is bigger than 4 centimetres in diameter, surgical treatment to remove it and to treat endometriosis will improve the chance of pregnancy.

Small cysts (2–4 centimetres) can be managed on a wait and see basis. Ovarian cysts are rarely cancerous, but this should be considered, particularly in the older woman having fertility treatment.

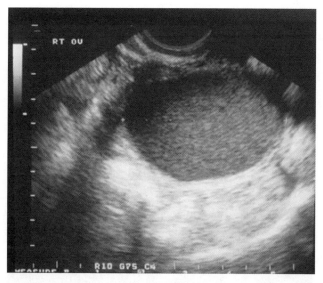

Figure 21.11 An endometrioma is filled with blood and has a typical 'ground glass' appearance on scan. Reproduced from Serhal. P., and Overton. O., *Good Clinical Practice in Assisted Reproduction* (2004), pp 226–55, with permission from Cambridge University Press.

Endometrial polyps

These are small skin tags found within the lining of the womb. Small polyps just a few millimetres in diameter are probably not significant. Larger polyps are thought to affect fertility by acting as a 'coil'.

Polyps can cause symptoms of irregular bleeding, particularly bleeding between the periods. They are commonly found during investigations such as hysterosalpingogram or ultrasound scan.

Removal is normally advised. A small telescope is passed through the cervix and the polyp picked off or shaved off (resected) using a heated wire. This operation, which is called a polypectomy, can be carried out under a local or general anaesthetic as a day case.

Whatever the problem, you may need time to make a decision and should have time to reflect and ask more questions.

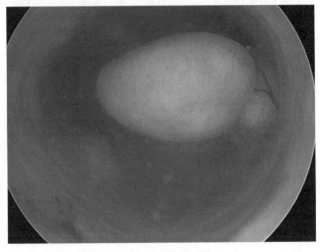

Figure 21.12 An endometrial polyp seen at hysteroscopy

22

Tubal surgery

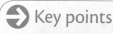

> **Key points**
>
> * Blocked Fallopian tubes are successfully opened in about eight out of ten operations but the pregnancy rate is much lower than this.
> * The risk of ectopic pregnancy is as high as 1 in 10.
> * About one in seven women get pregnant within 12 months after tubal surgery.

Tubal damage and adhesions (scarring) usually happen because of past infection. This could be a sexually transmitted infection or infection after miscarriage or childbirth, appendicitis, or abdominal surgery. The infection can cause blockage of the tubes anywhere along their length, as well as adhesions wrapping around the ovaries and tubes. The egg becomes trapped in these cobweb-like adhesions and cannot reach the Fallopian tube.

Tubal surgery to open the tubes and/or release adhesions may be possible. The tubes are examined to see how much they have been affected. Laparoscopy looks at the outside of the tubes, and hysterosalpingography (HSG) looks at the inside or lining of the tubes. The chance of pregnancy after tubal surgery depends on the woman's age (her 'biological clock'), the presence of any male factor, and the extent of the damage. If there is a sperm problem or the woman is over 37 years old, IVF offers a better chance of pregnancy. IVF collects the eggs directly from the ovaries, and so the tubes are 'bypassed'. It also allows several eggs to be collected, some for replacement and others for storage.

Blocked tubes (hydrosalpinges)

Hydrosalpinx (from 'hydro' = water and 'salpinx' = tube) is the name given to tubes that are blocked and filled with fluid. If tubal surgery has already been tried but the tubes have closed up again, or if the tubes are so badly damaged that tubal

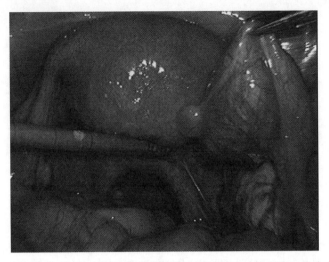

Figure 22.1 Hydrosalpinx: a blocked tube filled with fluid. Reproduced from Serhal and Overton, *Good Clinical Practice in Assisted Reproduction* (2004), with permission of Cambridge University Press.

surgery is not an option, removal of the damaged tubes (salpingectomy) may be discussed. Removal of such badly damaged tubes seems to improve the success rate of IVF treatment.

However, many questions remain unclear, especially how to decide which women would benefit from salpingectomy. The general consensus is that if the tubes are so damaged that the hydrosalpinx can be seen on scan, salpingectomy would improve pregnancy rates in IVF. Deciding how badly the tubes are damaged is the key question, and removing the tubes without careful consideration is certainly not the answer. Doctors have different opinions in how to treat damaged tubes.

Salpingostomy

If the tubes are blocked at the very end, it may be possible to open them by an operation called salpingostomy. During the operation, any scar tissue covering the end of the tube is removed. The tube is opened and turned back on itself (like a cuff) so that it will remain open (Figure 22.2).

Salpingostomy is usually carried out under a general anaesthetic, either through a bikini line cut or laparoscopically. It is normal to feel uncomfortable after the operation, and regular painkillers are prescribed. Antibiotics are also given to prevent any further infection following the surgery. How long you need to stay in hospital varies: it can be as short as 24 hours for keyhole surgery, or a few days with a traditional operation. You will be able to go home as soon as you can eat and drink, walk around, and pass urine. You will be able to go back to work about a month later depending on the job you do.

170

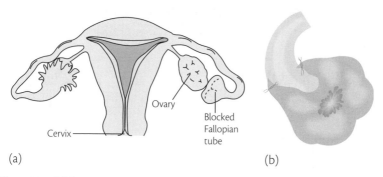

(a)   (b)

Figure 22.2 Salpingostomy: an operation to unblock the tubes. (b) close-up the opened tube.

How successful is salpingostomy?

The tubes can be opened successfully in 80 per cent of cases, but only about 15 per cent of women will get pregnant in the 12 months after the operation. Successful treatment means that a woman may be able to achieve more than one natural pregnancy. The operation is effective immediately, and you should start having sexual intercourse again as soon as you are comfortable (there is no need to wait for your follow-up appointment). The highest chance of getting pregnant is in the first 6 months after surgery. This is because adhesions can re-form or the tube can close up again.

- Tubes are successfully opened in eight out of ten operations.
- One in seven women become pregnant in the 12 months after surgery.
- One in ten of the pregnancies will be ectopic.

The chance of natural pregnancy and pregnancy after IVF is reduced if one or both tubes are a hydrosalpinx. Exactly why is not known, but suggestions are that it affects how the tube works and that the fluid within the tubes affects the swimming ability of the sperm and may have a 'poisonous' effect on the forming embryo.

Are there any alternative treatments for hydrosalpinx?

Salpingectomy may have an adverse effect on the blood supply around the ovaries and most doctors now advise clipping the tube rather than salpingectomy.

Other treatments have been tried. Needle drainage of the fluid within the hydrosalpinx is unsuccessful as fluid re-accumulates within 2 days. Tubal catheterization has been suggested as an alternative, but there are no published results

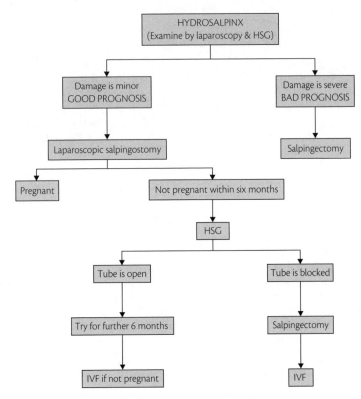

Figure 22.3 Management of hydrosalpinx

to show how effective it is and whether the risk of infection is increased. Another option is needle drainage of the hydrosalpinx at the time of egg retrieval.

Tubal catheterization

If the tubes are blocked where they join the uterus (womb), then treatment may be possible by selective salpingography. Similar to HSG, a small catheter or wire is passed through the cervix to try and reopen the tubes. In one study the tubes were successfully opened in 70–90 per cent of women, with pregnancy rates of 12–36 per cent. In 2 per cent of women, the guide wire perforated the tube, but there were no serious side effects. Ectopic pregnancy occurred in 3 per cent of women. If treatment does not result in a pregnancy, tubal surgery or IVF is still possible.

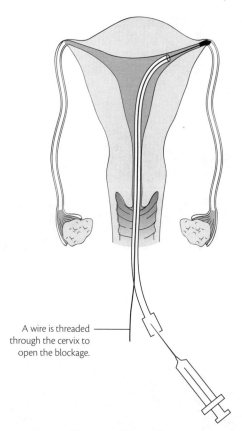

A wire is threaded through the cervix to open the blockage.

Figure 22.4 Selective salpingography can be used to try and unblock the tubes.

Adhesiolysis

Adhesions are scar tissue that forms between the internal organs, causing them to stick together. Adhesions around the tubes and ovaries trap the egg and prevent pregnancy. They can be fine, like cobwebs, or dense so that insides are 'glued' together. Adhesions can result from infection or previous surgery, but may also be caused by endometriosis.

Adhesiolysis is a major operation, usually carried out under general anaesthetic either through a bikini line cut or laparoscopically using 'keyhole surgery'. The adhesions are released using special instruments.

It is normal to feel uncomfortable after the operation, and regular painkillers are prescribed. Antibiotics are also given to prevent any further infection following the surgery. How long you need to stay in hospital varies: it can be as short

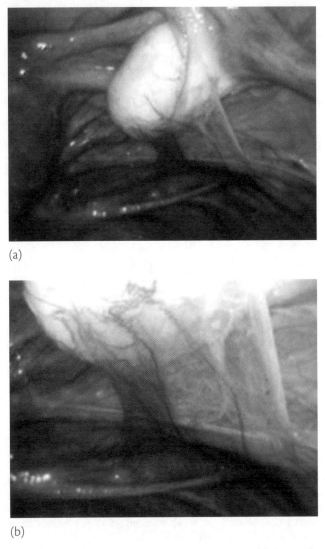

(a)

(b)

Figure 22.5 Adhesions form between different parts of the body. (a) shows adhesions around the ovary and (b) a close-up view.

as 24 hours for keyhole surgery, or a few days with a traditional operation. You will be able to go home as soon as you can eat and drink, walk around, and pass urine. You will be able to go back to work about a month later depending on the job you do.

How successful is adhesiolysis?

In young women, with no male factor fertility, the success of tubal surgery is a 15 per cent pregnancy rate over 12 months i.e. three women out of twenty will get pregnant over 12 months of trying. Successful treatment means that a woman may be able to achieve more than one natural pregnancy. The operation is effective immediately and you should start having sexual intercourse again as soon as you are comfortable (there is no need to wait for your follow-up appointment). The highest chance of getting pregnant is in the first 6 months after surgery. This is because adhesions can re-form.

What are the risks of tubal surgery?

Bowel damage

Adhesions bind structures together, and so bowel can be wrapped up in the adhesions. If it is anticipated that the bowel is involved, you may be given a strong laxative before the operation to clean out the bowel. The bowel is carefully unpicked and released. Great care is taken not to damage the bowel. If damage does occur, the bowel will need to be repaired. It would be usual to call a bowel surgeon to repair the bowel.

Ectopic pregnancy

Infection may have damaged other parts of the tube. By surgically opening the tubes, you may increase your chance of having an ectopic pregnancy (pregnancy in the tube), which can be life-threatening. The chance of an ectopic pregnancy may be as high as one in ten pregnancies. For this reason, you are advised to have a scan when you are 6 weeks pregnant (sooner if you are in pain) to check that the pregnancy has reached the lining of the womb.

23

Reversal of sterilization and reversal of vasectomy

Key points

◆ About 3% to 5% of women who have undergone tubal sterilization express regret and request reversal of sterilization. A similar percentage of men decide to have their vasectomies reversed.

◆ Reversal of sterilization is a major surgical procedure involving tubal surgery.

◆ The pregnancy rate following microsurgery for reversal of sterilization over 12 months is 70% to 80% i.e. seven out of ten women will be pregnant after 12 months of trying.

Reversal of sterilization

There are different ways to sterilize the tubes. Whether it is possible to 'reverse the sterilization' depends on how the sterilization was done, particularly on how much of the Fallopian tubes has been damaged.

The most common method in the UK is to sterilize the tubes by placing a clip or ring over the tube. This is the most reversible method, as little of the tube is damaged. The portion of the tube under the clip dies, so reversal is not simply removing the clips. The damaged part of the tube needs to be cut out and the two ends rejoined. Other methods of sterilization include cauterization (diathermy) or cutting of the tubes. Unless accurate surgical notes can be obtained, a laparoscopy is needed to see how much of the tube remains and where the tube has been sterilized. X-rays (hysterosalpingography) may also be helpful.

❌ **Myth:** Reversal of sterilization can be done by just undoing the clips.

❗ **Fact:** Reversal of sterilization is a major operation involving tubal surgery

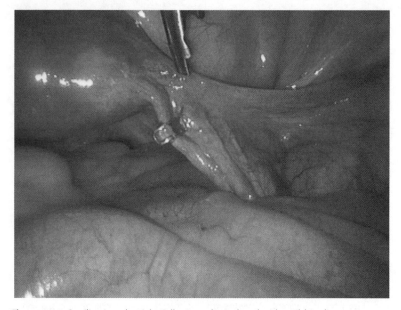

Figure 23.1 Sterilization: the right Fallopian tube is closed with a Filshie clip.

About 3–5 per cent of women who have had tubal sterilization express regret and request reversal of sterilization. The first step is to check the sperm sample of the partner in order to prevent later disappointment for the couple. This is particularly important if he has not had any children.

Pre-pregnancy considerations

Before going ahead with reversal of sterilization, you and your doctor should think about your health if you do get pregnant (see Chapter 2).

- Get as fit as you can.
- Give up smoking.
- Reduce weight or put on weight if you need to.
- Check with your doctor that you are immune to rubella (german measles).
- Start taking folic acid tablets.
- Have a check-up with your doctor for any health problems that would affect you and/or a pregnancy (e.g. diabetes or high blood pressure).
- Check with your doctor to see if you are you taking any medicines that might affect the pregnancy and need to be changed before you get pregnant
- Tell your doctor if you have had problems in previous pregnancies, such as a weak cervix, that will need treatment during the pregnancy

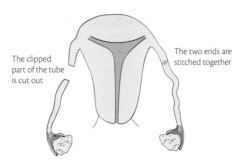

Figure 23.2 Reversal of sterilization.

Reversal of sterilization is usually carried out under a general anaesthetic either through a bikini line cut or laparoscopically by 'keyhole surgery'. A microscope is used to accurately cut out the blocked portion of the tubes and rejoin the ends. It is normal to feel uncomfortable after the operation, and regular pain-killers are prescribed. Antibiotics are also given to prevent any further infection following the surgery. Pain after the operation is normal. Complications of surgery are bruising, infection in the stitches, and, later, adhesions and stricture (narrowing) of the rejoined tubes.

How long you need to stay in hospital varies; it can be as short as 24 hours for keyhole surgery, or a few days with a traditional operation. You will be able to go home as soon as you can eat and drink, pass urine, and walk around, and your pain is manageable with painkillers. You will be able to go back to work about a month later depending on the job you do.

How successful is reversal of sterilization?

Microsurgery (operating with the use of a microscope) for reversal of sterilization is very successful where there has been little damage to the tubes (e.g. clips). The pregnancy rate over 12 months is 70–80 per cent. Where diathermy has been used to sterilise the tubes, reversal is less successful because more of the tube has been destroyed.

Successful treatment means that a woman may be able to achieve more than one natural pregnancy. The operation is effective immediately and you should start having sexual intercourse again as soon as you are comfortable (there is no need to wait for your follow-up appointment). The highest chance of getting pregnant is in the first 6 months after surgery. This is because adhesions can re-form or the join can narrow or block (stricture).

Ectopic pregnancy

Scar tissue at the site of the join can result in an increased chance of ectopic pregnancy (pregnancy in the tube), which can be life-threatening. The chance of an ectopic pregnancy may be as high as one in ten pregnancies. For this reason we advise you to have a scan when you are 6 weeks pregnant (sooner if you are in pain) to check that the pregnancy has reached the uterus (womb).

Reversal of vasectomy

Approximately 3–5 per cent of men decide to have their vasectomy reversed. There are many reasons why men wish to have theis done, although commonly the man has met a new partner. Your vasectomy can be reversed by an operation (surgical reversal) or test tube techniques can be used to obtain sperm directly from the testis for IVF and ICSI (see Chapter 14)

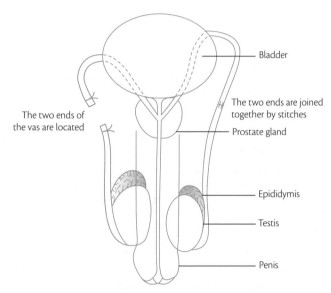

Figure 23.3 Reversal of vasectomy.

The choice of operation, i.e. sperm retrieval or reversal, mainly depends upon the wishes of the patient and the time elapsed since the vasectomy was performed. The age of the female partner is also very important, as there are fewer chances that a vasectomy reversal will work as the female gets older.

Technique

Surgical reversal of vasectomy should be carried out using microsurgical techniques (operating with the use of a microscope). However, some surgeons argue that using a loupe or special magnifying spectacles is just as good. In 30 per cent of cases a more complex join will need to be performed between the epididymis and vas deferens; this is called a vaso-epididostomy. This can only be decided by the surgeon at the time of surgery. Surgery is usually performed under a general anaesthetic and takes 2–3 hours. The type of incision used largely depends upon the preference of the surgeon, but will either be on the scrotum or occasionally in the groin area. At the same time as performing the join, sperm can also be taken from the testicle and frozen. This could be used if surgery to reverse the vasectomy is not possible or if the vasectomy reversal is not successful.

The blocked portion of the tube is cut out and the two ends are stitched together using very fine suture material. Antibiotics are given at the time of operation to prevent infection.

A semen analysis is usually performed 6 weeks to 3 months after surgery, although it may take up to 6 months before sperm appears in the ejaculate.

Complications of surgery are pain and bruising, infection in the stitches in the early days after surgery and later of sperm granuloma, and stricture (narrowing of the rejoined segment of the tube). Occasionally damage or atrophy to the testicle can occur, and the testicle can shrink and become small.

Success rates

Successful treatment means that a man may be able to father more than one natural pregnancy. As with reversal of female sterilization, the operation is effective immediately and you should start having sexual intercourse again as soon as you are comfortable. The highest chance of getting pregnant is in the first 6 months after surgery.

Success rates for reversal of vasectomy depend on how long ago the vasectomy was done, the type of procedure performed, and the technical expertise of the surgeon. This is because anti-sperm antibodies develop and affect the motility of the sperm and their ability to fertilize an egg. The longer the time since the vasectomy, the more anti-sperm antibodies there will be. There will also be more scarring with time.

Test tube techniques

If the female partner is older or the vasectomy was performed a long time ago, patients may be advised to have sperm retrieval and ICSI. There are a variety of ways of obtaining sperm (see Chapter 10).

Table 23.1 Success rates for reversal of vasectomy

Time since vasectomy	Sperm present (%)	Pregnancy rate (%)
Less than 3 years	97	76
3–8 years	88	53
9–14 years	79	44
More than 15 years	71	30

These results should be compared with the IVF success rate of 28% nationally per attempt.

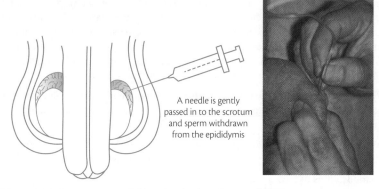

A needle is gently passed in to the scrotum and sperm withdrawn from the epididymis

Figure 23.4 Percutaneous epididymal aspiration of sperm (PESA).

Percutaneous epididymal aspiration of sperm (PESA)

Sperm can be recovered from the epididymis as an alternative to reversal of vasectomy. Under local anaesthetic, a needle is passed through the skin of the scrotum into the epididymis and sperm are retrieved. There are few complications and the procedure is not too uncomfortable. Fewer sperm are recovered and therefore it is necessary to combine this technique with a cycle of ICSI. Sometimes, only poor-quality sperm or no sperm are obtained, and a cut may need to be made on the testicle and other techniques, such as MESA and TESE (see Chapter 10), will need to be used.

Each sperm is injected directly into the egg. The success rate is approximately 28 per cent per cycle of treatment, but is proportional to the woman's age. The success rate for women over 40 is 10 per cent.

 Personal history

William and Joanne wanted to start a family together. William had been married before and, after two children, had had a vasectomy. They discussed the options of donor insemination, but wanted to have a biological child together. William had surgery to reverse his vasectomy and at the same time sperm were recovered from the epididymis (MESA) and frozen. After 12 months, pregnancy hadn't happened naturally. The stored sperm were used for ICSI and Joanne was happily pregnant after the second attempt.

24

Pregnancy after fertility treatment

> ## ➔ Key points
>
> ◆ In early pregnancy, it is recommended that women stop drinking alcohol and smoking and reduce their intake of caffeine.
>
> ◆ Approximately one in six pregnancies is lost in the first 3 months. Miscarriage is more common in older women and may be more common in women with PCOS.
>
> ◆ There is no increased risk of miscarriage following fertility treatment compared with natural conception.
>
> ◆ Ectopic pregnancy occurs in approximately one in 20 pregnancies following fertility treatment.
>
> ◆ Fertility treatment can result in multiple births; approximately 25 per cent of IVF pregnancies result in twins. Multiple pregnancy carries risks for both mother and babies.

Congratulations! That positive pregnancy test makes all the investigations and treatment worthwhile. Pregnancy tests bought over the counter for home use are very accurate. They measure a hormone called beta-HCG, which is only made by the developing pregnancy. It can be detected in the urine from about 10 days after conception, and tests become reliable 14 days after conception. The clinic will advise you on which day you should do your test; some clinics confirm it on a blood sample.

The fertility clinic will offer you an ultrasound scan in early pregnancy. This is usually done at 7 weeks gestation (5 weeks after egg collection or insemination). At this stage an embryo and heartbeat can usually be seen. Multiple pregnancy can be detected. Ectopic (tubal) pregnancy is uncommon but may be diagnosed.

The first 3 months

In early pregnancy it is advisable to stop drinking alcohol and, of course, to stop smoking. Reduce your intake of caffeine in coffee, tea, and soft drinks.

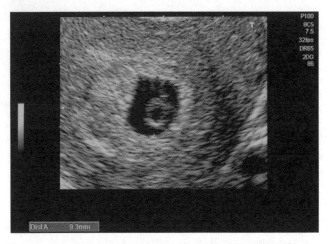

Figure 24.1 Ultrasound scan of a 5-week pregnancy with yolk sac (food for the developing fetus).

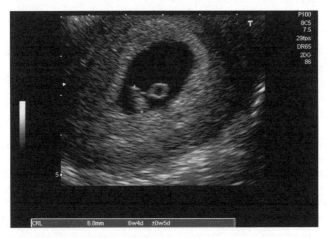

Figure 24.2 Ultrasound scan of a 6-week pregnancy.

You should try to eat a balanced diet with plenty of vegetables and fruit. However, many women experience morning sickness (which can last all day) and often find that small meals of carbohydrate such as toast or digestive biscuits are the easiest to take. Don't worry too much if you are unable to eat properly at this time, as it will not harm the pregnancy. Drink enough fluids, and see your doctor if your sickness is severe.

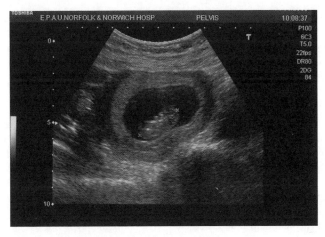

Figure 24.3 Ultrasound scan of an 8-week pregnancy.

Folic acid supplements should be taken before pregnancy and carried on for the first 3 months of pregnancy. Folic acid reduces the chance of having a baby with serious abnormalities of the nervous system such as spina bifida. The recommended dose is 400 micrograms daily (this is the standard dose in over-the-counter pregnancy supplements). Some women prefer to take a multi-vitamin tablet—choose one designed for pregnancy, because these contain folic acid and not too much vitamin A (which can be harmful in excess).

Exercise in pregnancy can be a controversial subject. Exercise should be avoided around the time of egg collection and embryo transfer. Most fertility clinics advise against exercise in the early weeks of pregnancy, but you do not have to be a couch potato either. Avoid strenuous exercise or potentially dangerous sports such as horse-riding, but walking the dog, swimming, or gentle yoga are safe.

Sex is best avoided immediately after embryo transfer, as the ovaries may be tender and swollen for several weeks after IVF. Sex does not cause miscarriage, but should be avoided if there is any bleeding.

Medicines in pregnancy

Medicines should be kept to a minimum in pregnancy, but several common medicines have been used for years and are considered safe in pregnancy. If you need to take a painkiller, choose paracetamol. Several types of antibiotics, including penicillin, can be used. You should tell your doctor that you are pregnant even if you consult him/her for another problem.

If you have been prescribed hormone supplements (usually progesterone) after IVF treatment, you will need to keep taking these for the first few weeks of pregnancy. It is safe to stop by 12 weeks. Hormone supplements are vital for egg donation pregnancies, but can still be stopped at around 12 weeks.

Some women will be prescribed aspirin in early pregnancy, and this is considered safe. Heparin injections to reduce blood clotting have no known effect on the developing pregnancy, although there are possible side effects for the mother. Steroid tablets and intravenous immunoglobulin (IVIG) have no proven benefit in early pregnancy and have potential risks, so they should not be used.

Travelling in pregnancy

It may be best to avoid travelling, unless essential, in the early weeks of pregnancy. It is not harmful, but it can be tiring and stressful. Flying in pressurized aircraft should not affect the pregnancy. Long-distance air travel carries a small risk of thrombosis (blood clots) for pregnant women, and you should take precautions against this. It is unwise to travel far from home in the last 2 months of pregnancy, and indeed airlines will not accept women passengers in late pregnancy. If you are planning to travel abroad in pregnancy, think about your destination—could you get medical help if an emergency arises? Pregnancy is not the time for a holiday 'getting away from it all' in a remote destination far from medical care!

Miscarriage

There is no greater risk of miscarriage after fertility treatment than after natural conception. About one in six pregnancies are lost in the first 3 months. Miscarriage is more common in older mothers, and may be more common in women with polycystic ovary syndrome.

Often an ultrasound scan gives the first sign that the pregnancy is not growing and might miscarry. Sometimes bleeding or pain is the first sign. Very early miscarriage (5–7 weeks) is like a late heavy period and usually requires no treatment. Miscarriage at 8–12 weeks may need hospital admission and a minor operation to empty the womb (ERPC, 'evacuation of retained products of conception'). However many miscarriages come away naturally, and the clinic will use ultrasound to check that the womb is empty.

If miscarriage occurs repeatedly, further tests should be offered to see if any cause can be found which could be treatable. However, most miscarriages are caused by a genetic problem in the developing embryo which is a 'one-off' event, and the outlook for the next pregnancy is good.

Ectopic pregnancy

This means a pregnancy growing outside the womb, usually in the Fallopian tube. It is not common, affecting one in 100 pregnancies in the UK, but is more likely to occur in women who have had infertility problems, especially if the tubes are damaged or scarred. About one in 20 pregnancies after fertility treatment are ectopic.

Ectopic pregnancy is usually picked up early in women who have had fertility treatment. It may be suspected when ultrasound shows no pregnancy sac developing in the womb, despite a strongly positive pregnancy test in a blood sample. It is sometimes visible on ultrasound.

Ectopic pregnancy is dangerous because the pregnancy may rupture through the Fallopian tube and cause heavy internal bleeding. The first signs may be pain in the lower abdomen and faintness; if not detected, bleeding may be life-threatening. These complications do not usually occur before 7 weeks' gestation. Ectopic pregnancy is usually treated by surgery. The damaged tube usually needs to be removed by laparoscopy (keyhole surgery). A small early ectopic pregnancy may also be treated by medication, using methotrexate injection; this avoids removing the tube but takes a few weeks to resolve.

Women who have a rhesus-negative blood group should be given 'anti-D' if they have surgical treatment for miscarriage or ectopic pregnancy. This is a blood product, given as a single dose by injection, which prevents the body from reacting to 'foreign' blood cells from the pregnancy. If sensitivity to rhesus-positive blood occurs, it may complicate future pregnancies.

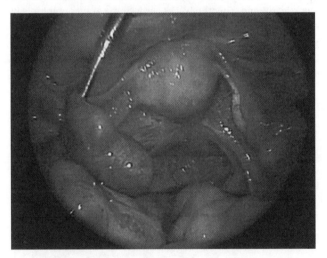

Figure 24.4 Laparoscopy of an ectopic pregnancy.

Antenatal care

After the first 3 months of pregnancy, your medical care will be taken over by the antenatal clinic. Once the pregnancy is confirmed, you will need to decide, with advice from your GP and fertility clinic, where you would like to deliver your baby. In the UK, almost all women have NHS care during pregnancy, even if they have been private patients for fertility treatment.

The antenatal clinic will check routine blood tests, including screening you for anaemia, and offer you at least one further ultrasound scan at 18–20 weeks which checks the baby's development. All women in the UK are offered screening tests for Down syndrome during pregnancy.

Your check-ups during pregnancy are usually shared between the hospital, your GP, and your local midwife. If complications occur, you will be referred to the hospital consultant. Assisted conception pregnancies are more likely to need hospital care, mainly because mothers are likely to be older and there are many twin pregnancies.

Multiple pregnancy

Fertility treatment can result in multiple birth; currently one in four IVF pregnancies are twins. A small number of triplet or even quadruplet pregnancies can also result from fertility drug treatment. If you are carrying twins or more, you will need special care in pregnancy. You should plan to deliver in a hospital that has facilities to care for small babies.

The biggest risk with multiple pregnancy is prematurity. On average, twins are born 3 weeks early, and triplets 6 weeks early. Some of these multiple births will occur so early that the babies need intensive care, and some babies may not survive, or will grow up with disabilities.

Because of these risks, you may be offered selective termination (also called fetal reduction) for multiple pregnancies of triplets or more to reduce the

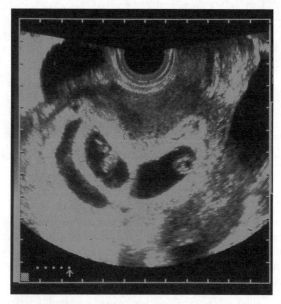

Figure 24.5 Ultrasound scan of a multiple pregnancy.

pregnancy to twins. This is done by injecting one of the pregnancy sacs under ultrasound guidance. Selective termination is usually done at 10–12 weeks; before this, it is quite possible that the pregnancy will reduce naturally. There is a small risk that the procedure will cause the whole pregnancy to miscarry, but this needs to be balanced against the risks of continuing with the multiple pregnancies. Having wanted a baby so much, this can be heart-breaking. This is why fertility treatment aims to avoid multiple pregnancy.

You are more likely to experience complications of pregnancy, such as severe morning sickness, high blood pressure, and diabetes, with twins or triplets. Most multiple pregnancies need delivery by Caesarean section, which carries more risk for the mother than a normal birth.

Pregnancy and older mothers

Many women who conceive after suffering from infertility have spent years trying for a child, and they tend to be older than other mothers. Unfortunately, this puts them at higher risk of miscarriage and pregnancy complications. There is also an increased chance of having a baby with abnormalities, and many couples choose to have special tests in pregnancy. Remember, though, that the great majority of pregnancies end happily in the safe delivery of a healthy baby!

Pregnancy in older mothers is discussed in more detail in Chapter 20.

Children born after fertility treatment

When IVF was developed in the 1970s there was a great deal of concern that this technology might cause abnormalities, but these fears were unfounded. Many thousands of IVF children have been followed up without showing an increased risk of abnormalities. Indeed, the first IVF baby, Louise Brown, is now married and a mother herself, perhaps the ultimate proof.

Embryo freezing has also given rise to thousands of healthy children over the last 15–20 years. More recent techniques are less well studied because fewer children have been born and they are still young. For example, egg freezing has only led to a few hundred pregnancies around the world. Studies on animals have been useful—techniques are often developed in mice and sheep, and IVF and insemination techniques are used in veterinary medicine—but studying animals cannot compare with the complexity of children's development. Two techniques, in particular, are under the spotlight.

ICSI (intra-cytoplasmic sperm injection) (see Chapter 14) is now a common technique and highly successful, but there have been concerns that injecting the sperm deep into the egg could damage the egg's genetic material. Also, ICSI can be carried out with sperm that are not healthy enough to fertilize the egg naturally. Studies of children born following ICSI have suggested a slight increase in the risk of rare genetic abnormalities. Some men with very low sperm counts have a genetic reason for infertility, such as loss of genes on the Y chromosome, which can be passed on to their sons.

Embryo biopsy involves taking one or two cells away from the early embryo (see Chapter 16). The embryo is still able to develop and implant, and pregnancy rates are not reduced, but we do not yet have enough information about the children born from this technique. Therefore it is sensible to use this new technology only when necessary, when there is a significant risk of a child being born with a serious genetic disorder.

Children born after fertility treatment have also been followed up to see whether they are socially disadvantaged. These studies are very reassuring. These children are usually growing up in loving and stable families; indeed their parents are less likely to separate than other couples. Parents may be over-protective towards a child who has been so badly wanted, and many grow up as only children, which can be a mixed blessing. There has been particular focus on children born to same-sex couples and to single women. Again, the follow-up studies are reassuring and these children do not seem to be disadvantaged. This supports the wider availability of fertility treatment for same-sex couples and single women. Usually these children grow up aware of their genetic origin and their mother's treatment with donor insemination; however, not all heterosexual couples tell their children that they were conceived by gamete donation. Couples are more likely to be open about egg donation, where the mother has carried and given birth to the child, than sperm donation where the father has no biological link to the child. The psychological evidence suggests that children can cope with this knowledge and that honesty is better than secrecy, as unexpected disclosure can be very traumatic.

Case study

Razia was thrilled when she became pregnant. She had gone through IVF with ICSI because her husband's sperm count was low. At the first scan she was delighted to be told she was carrying twins. Shortly afterwards, she developed terrible morning sickness and had to take 2 weeks off work. By 4 months of pregnancy she was feeling better, and proud of her visible 'bump'.

At 26 weeks of pregnancy, Razia woke up one morning feeling wet and was shocked to see a bloodstain on the bed. Her husband called an ambulance and she was taken to the maternity unit, where a scan showed that the placenta (afterbirth) of one of the twins was lying low in the womb. She was allowed home 2 days later but didn't go back to work. Her family did everything for her to allow her to rest.

At 32 weeks, she had more bleeding. She was admitted to hospital and given steroid injections to help the babies' lungs to mature; she was told that emergency delivery might be needed. Fortunately, the bleeding settled, but Razia stayed in hospital and, as the placenta was still covering the entrance of the womb, her consultant advised her to have a Caesarean section.

The twins were delivered at 34 weeks. Razia couldn't see them at once, as they were in the Special Care Baby Unit, but her husband took photos and she visited them as soon as she could get out of bed after the operation. The midwives helped her to express some breast milk, and the babies thrived. After 3 weeks the twins came home—looking after them took every minute of the day, but Razia felt that her life was complete.

25

Coping with infertility

> ## Key points
>
> ◆ People with fertility problems may find they are having to cope with one of the hardest experiences of their lives.
>
> ◆ It is important to find what ways of coping suit you, not feel there is a right way to get through the uncertainty of treatment or the certainty of ending treatment.
>
> ◆ Forewarned is forearmed. It helps to get clued up to feel more in control.
>
> ◆ There are many different ways of coping. Couples may find they will do things differently and it helps to be able to discuss needs.
>
> ◆ The ending of treatment and facing life without your own children is a bereavement.

There is a lot to cope with

You have been told that there are fertility problems, although you have probably suspected that already. You now realize that you are going to need assisted reproductive technology if you are going to have a child and your world is suddenly changed; your relationships with your partner and family may be altered, your sense of yourself can feel damaged, your competent working self might feel like a failure, your future might not be what you had thought it would be, and you are looking at a life that feels completely different from anything you had hoped for or wanted. You are dealing with one of the hardest things anyone has to face.

Feeling despairing and overwhelmed is very, very painful but it is absolutely normal. Many people, having had a shocking experience, seem to feel that there must be a 'right' way of dealing with it and that they don't know what it is. 'Coping' is very culturally determined and nobody wants to be seen as not coping within their own social setting. For instance, you can see loud and dramatic mourning in other cultures which, if seen in the UK, would be described as 'not coping'.

There isn't a right way

For you, there is your way and this chapter is to help you think about it. Sometimes it is hard to think when overwhelmed by emotions.

The first coping mechanisms you will want to think about are those that will keep you going during the uncertainty, fear, and anxiety of not getting pregnant and the treatment that you've been advised you need to have a baby. Secondly, how do you cope if you reach the sad certainty of the failure of the treatment and you are reaching the conclusion that you will not be having your own child.

Forewarned is forearmed

During the process of investigations and treatment, it really does help you feel in control if you learn what's going on. Medical jargon can seem impenetrable, but if you know, for instance, what FSH stands for, then you feel more able to have a conversation with the doctor and less like someone who is being told what is going to be done to them. This decreases anxiety.

Websites are one of the best sources of information, but be careful not to be overwhelmed by miracle workers or information overload; go to the recognized sites of well-known support organizations or those that are recommended by your clinic, your counsellor, or your GP.

If you are the kind of person who feels better sharing fears and anxieties, then chat rooms (handle with care) and support groups are available.

The nurses at the clinic are probably able to give you more time than the consultants, so take it!

If you are provided with realistic information about what to expect from the actual experience of the procedure (e.g. 'your bladder will feel like it is bursting') as well as what the results of the test will reveal, this also helps to reduce stress.

Look at books; choose one whose style suits you (it may be this one!).

Write down the list of questions you want answered when you go for an appointment; even make notes while you are there. Being anxious plays havoc with your memory!

Support

Some people find support counselling really helpful; here you can give vent to your feelings without worrying that you might be upsetting the very people you need to help you. You can also explore particular aspects of your own history that may be adding to the stress during treatment. Uncovering some of these hidden stressors, for example guilt around an earlier termination or an unconscious attempt to replace a sibling lost when you were young, can be very liberating.

Mind/body relaxation techniques

Another tried and trusted coping strategy is learning some sort of mind/body relaxation technique. Some infertility counsellors run groups that offer this, which also have the added benefit of listening to other people's stories and how they cope. Again, this will be very much a matter of personal choice and you might be surprised, as a 'facts' person, finding yourself in the more alternative area of therapies.

Classes in yoga or meditation, where you are just another member of the class, not there for any other reason than to benefit from the liberation that deep concentration and focus can give, may help. For you, this might be liberation from the sometimes ceaseless gnawing away at the 'infertility issues' that fills up much of your waking or sleepless hours.

Men and women tend to cope differently

If you are able to have a quiet discussion about this difference with your partner so that you are both aware of the different coping mechanisms you use, this could prevent a lot of heartache.

Very generally, women tend to show and feel more anxiety and distress, whereas men tend to use strategies that keep emotions well controlled or sometimes displaced (e.g. taking out anger about the situation somewhere that has nothing to do with the problem, such as the supermarket check-out) and by being pragmatic and problem-solving (e.g. 'We'll just do IVF then, no point worrying about what we can't alter …'). The woman can experience this as unemotional and insensitive, when she is feeling that her body is failing her. She might want a discussion and reassurance to regain a sense of herself as a functioning and attractive woman when he might feel that focusing on something completely different for a bit would be better.

If you can try to take responsibility for your needs (which can be difficult when you feel so out of control) and share these with your partner as well as trying to hear what they need, then this does help you to feel effective. Does having a soothing massage help? Going to a football match? Watching something mindless on TV? Not going to baby-centred events? Going for long walks? Getting a pet? (Don't dismiss this as an obvious baby substitute; looking after something else is rewarding in itself and has been shown to reduce stress levels.) Doing something you've been postponing for years—salsa classes, cake decoration, getting fit, Thai boxing, changing your hair colour? Doing more of something you are good at? Sorting this out both quietly on your own and between the two of you can be therapeutic, revealing, and a really good beginning to a life together that may be without children, but also a good foundation for sharing needs when or if there is a baby, whose needs will be paramount.

All these strategies will of course be around when you have to face the finality of the end of treatment and that there will be no child of your own. You might be considering adoption, but first it is important that you are able to mourn the child you will never have.

This is bereavement

This bereavement is facing the loss of 'you as mother' or 'you as father' or 'us as parents' to your own child. When someone dies, even though it may be shocking and very sad, it is a sort of shared event, insofar as other people know about it and have some way of acknowledging the loss to a bereaved person. When you face this 'hidden' loss, you do not have that 'social safety net'.

First of all, remember that you have coped with problems before. Try to keep this in mind and you will find what is best for you. Although the problems were unlikely to have been as momentous as fertility problems and contemplating life without your own genetic child, the way you got through other difficulties will indicate that you already have ways of coping that work for you. Do you cry? Do you seek out friends? Do you run 10 miles or go to the gym? Do you shout at the dog or kick the door? Or go to bed? Watch the TV or race around tirelessly? Any of these reactions should give you some idea of how to cope with what is one of the most difficult challenges anyone has to face.

Crying must be the most appropriate reaction to grief, and yet so many people feel that this is a sign of 'not coping'. Some women in particular feel that if they start crying, the tears will never stop. This can feel so overwhelming that you may withdraw from social situations because you can't trust yourself not to break down. It is important to give yourself permission to do what gives you least stress. For example, for a while you don't attend child-oriented occasions, or gatherings where people ask THE question: 'Have you got children?'

Gradually, you will become more able to deal with these occasions, as your peer group moves into the next stage of parenting and you move on to different activities in your life. There will also be a more visible group of those who do not have children, whether out of choice or not, who will be doing some of the things that you are able to do with your unexpected life.

If you have tended to cope with difficulties by 'being busy' in any form that takes, you might seek out activities that will take your mind away from the grief, anger, jealousy, and maybe a sense of having failed in one of life's tasks. This is another coping mechanism and can work well, provided that somewhere you are aware that this is what all the activity is about. If you are really in a state of denial that you are actually dealing with an enormous loss in this particular and effective way for you, then there might be the danger of being 'caught unawares' by grief or even depression.

Self-help books, not specifically about infertility, can be a real help. You are a normal human being dealing with a real life crisis. The NHS self-help guides to Stress and Anxiety, Panic, Depression, and Low Mood are available from your GP. The Oxford Cognitive Therapy Centre do a series called 'Overcoming ...'.

Some of the topics they cover are Anxiety, Low Self-esteem, Social Anxiety, Depression, Mood Swings, Anger, and Irritability. Some primary care trusts make self-help books available on prescription. These are available from your library.

Again, a counsellor could offer you real help in coming to terms with the treatment failure and your loss. People who have been able to use some kind of therapeutic input have generally been able to adjust better to whatever kind of life they have chosen. Counselling is really helping you think through the process of coming to terms with the different future ahead of you—think about a new sense of purpose. Although this process might feel very lonely, others have walked this path too. Sometimes reading or listening to the experiences of others helps you to hear 'the still, sad music of humanity' (Wordsworth). *Beyond Childlessness*, by Rachel Black and Louise Scull, is a good example and offers ideas of how you might find some sense of meaning in the experience of infertility.

26

Adoption

→ Key points

◆ The average age of adoptive parents is 38 years.

◆ There is no official upper age limit for adopters, but most agencies require an age gap of no more than 40 years between child and adopter.

◆ There are very few babies under 1 year old available for adoption. This group only accounts for 1 per cent of adoptees.

◆ The average age of a child at adoption is a little over 4 years.

◆ Inter-country adoptions are becoming increasingly popular; more than 2200 children have been adopted from outside the UK since the year 2000.

Some would-be parents seek to adopt instead of undergoing fertility treatment, and others do so when treatment has been unsuccessful. There are many misperceptions surrounding adoption, particularly with regard to who is eligible to become an adopter and the backgrounds of children needing a new family.

The adopter profile

There are very few absolute requirements for the adopter, although a criminal record involving offences against children would exclude an individual from adopting a child. The interests of the child are always paramount, which includes finding a suitable placement within the minimal amount of time. The Adoption and Children Act 2002 has removed some of the previous restrictions for prospective adopters with the aim of enlarging the potential pool of adults who can provide a child with a loving and stable home.

Age

The average age of adoptive parents is 38 years. There is no official upper age limit for adopters, but most agencies work on an age gap of no more than about

40 years between child and adopter. Put another way, the adopter needs to be under the age of retirement whilst the child is at school.

Marital status

Marital status does not influence the chances of becoming an adoptive parent, although the vast majority of adopters (95 per cent) are married, with 92 per cent of the rest being female. Since January 2006, same-sex couples can jointly adopt under the Adoption and Children Act 2002. Previously this was only possible if one of the partnership adopted as a single parent, and therefore parental responsibility was not shared. The number of same-sex couples wishing to adopt or having completed the process successfully is not available at present.

Other children

Adopters may have other children or the adopted child may be their first. However, most adoption agencies require that the potential adopter is not having concurrent fertility treatment and some advocate waiting at least 6 months between stopping treatment and starting the application process.

Medical problems

The medical history of potential adopters is taken into account in the assessment process for adoption but, again, there are no absolute rules. The prospective parent(s) must have the energy to provide a nurturing environment suitable for a child of the age they wish to adopt and a reasonable lifespan expectation to go with this. Similarly, smoking is not an absolute bar to adoption, but being a smoker may place the potential adopter at a disadvantage because of the known associated health risks.

The adopted child

Over 60 000 children are in the care of local authorities in England and Wales, and just under 4000 of these children are adopted each year (excluding those adopted by relatives and step-parents). The majority of children who are adopted have been cared for in foster homes rather than institutions, although many have had several foster parents. With the exception of infants placed for adoption, most children spend over 3 years in care. Interestingly, there are slightly more boys in care than girls, but a majority of adopters prefer to adopt girls; however, almost equal numbers of boys and girls are actually adopted.

Very few babies under 1 year old are available for adoption; this group only accounts for 1 per cent of adoptees. The average age of a child at adoption is a little over 4 years. However, over a third are adopted with at least one sibling. The majority of children awaiting adoption were taken into the care of the local authority because of concerns for their well-being, and nearly half of those adopted have special needs.

Age at adoption

- The average age at adoption is 4 years 1 month
- 5 per cent (190) of children adopted during the year ending 31 March 2006 were under 1 year old.
- 64 per cent (2300) were aged between 1 and 4 years.
- 26 per cent (900) were aged between 5 and 9 years.
- 5 per cent (180) were aged between 10 and 15 years.

(Figures for England and Wales)

Ethnic background

Fortunately, it has been recognized that placing a child in a suitable loving home is the overriding priority, including for children from an ethnic minority background when there is no prospective adopter from an appropriate ethnic group. In fact, 90 per cent of adopted children are white, and three-quarters of those from an ethnic minority are of mixed parentage. Where there is no suitable prospective adopter from a similar ethnic background, a child from an ethnic minority will be placed with adoptive parent(s) who are prepared to support the child's cultural and ethnic identity.

The adoption process

Assessment and approval

The first step in the adoption process is to register with an adoption agency. It is usual to register with a local agency, although there may be particular reasons why you may prefer to register outside your region. It is possible to make initial enquiries with several agencies, although the actual application can only be submitted through one. Adoption agencies are run by either the local authority (Social Work Department in Scotland) or by a voluntary organization. It is possible to obtain a list of both types of adoption agency via associations such as the British Association for Adoption & Fostering (BAAF), Adoption UK, and the Consortium of Voluntary Adoption Agencies (see 'Useful addresses').

Once you have selected the agency, you need to submit a formal application to be assessed for adoption. The assessment process is lengthy (6–8 months), thorough, and considers all aspects of your life. During this time, and sometimes even before you have submitted your application, you will need to attend preparatory sessions which are aimed at helping you to be certain of your decision as well as understanding the assessment process. The sessions also help you to prepare to become adoptive parents, covering issues from helping a child to settle into the family to understanding the background and needs of an adopted child.

If you are adopting a child from the UK, there is no fee for any part of the application or assessment process. The assessment is carried out by a social worker from the agency. It includes personal questions including those on attitudes and beliefs, work/career plans, and social as well as financial circumstances. The social worker will visit you at home, usually six to eight times ('home visits') and you will have to see your GP for a medical. Personal checks will be carried out with your employer, the local authority, the Criminal Records Bureau (CRB) or Disclosure Scotland, and two or three personal referees. Many find this part of the process particularly difficult to cope with and very intrusive.

Once the assessment is complete, a written report will be prepared which will include a recommendation on the type of child/children you would best be able to provide a home for. The report will be presented to you and you will have 10 working days to comment on it before it goes to the adoption panel.

You will be invited to attend the adoption panel, which consists of approximately ten people, including social workers, medical and legal advisers, and lay members such as adopted adults. The panel will recommend a decision to the agency who are then responsible for your final approval to adopt. Over 90 per cent of applicants who are presented to the panel gain this approval. Of course, there are appeal processes should you not receive approval, but the agency has a duty to keep you informed of any reservations that might arise during the assessment and help you to improve your chances if this is possible.

Case study

Sarah and Marc had been trying to have a baby for 2½ years when Sarah was found to have blocked Fallopian tubes during fertility investigations. Although IVF may have helped them to conceive, the couple did not feel that the treatment was right for them and they preferred to adopt. However, the whole assessment process was very distressing for Marc, who found himself becoming defensive and argumentative during meetings with their social worker. The social worker put them in contact with another couple who had struggled similarly with the assessment process but now had successfully adopted a 3-year-old girl. This helped Marc to realize that the assessment was a standard process and that he was not being singled out. Marc and Sarah have now been approved as adoptive parents and have just been matched with 2-year-old twin boys.

Matching

Matching with a child can now begin. Initially, this is usually done with children who have a formal plan for adoption and are registered with the agency you have applied to. In England and Wales there is also a national register, the Adoption Register, to which children planned for adoption are referred.

The aim of the Adoption Register is to increase the chances of a child being matched with a suitable adopter, even if the match is not local. Children must be referred within 3 months of the formal decision that adoption is in the child's best interest. Similarly, approved adopters will be referred to the Adoption Register (with consent) within 3 months of receiving approval if a potential match is not being pursued. Potential adopters can be referred as soon as their approval is formalized if they so wish and with the consent of their agency. Between 100 and 150 children a year are matched with their new families in this way. At present, the Adoption Register does not cover Scotland, but there are other registers that do.

How the match is made

Up to five possible matches can be considered at any one time. The details of the adopter(s) and adoptee are exchanged between the respective social workers to consider the suitability of the match. You will also receive brief details of the child. If the match is considered viable by all concerned, detailed information will be forwarded. If the match still looks promising, you will usually receive a visit from the child's social worker at your home. At this stage, it is very common for several potential adopters to be interviewed. The final decision will be made according to the best interests of the child and will take into account all aspects of their life and background, including any wishes of the birth family.

Once all concerned agree to a potential match, a written adoption placement report is presented to an adoption panel, 10 days after you have been given a copy to comment on. The panel will make a recommendation to the child's adoption panel who will make the final decision regarding the placement.

Meeting your potential adoptive child

The child's social worker will arrange for you to meet the child once formal approval has been gained. The introduction will be appropriate to the child's age, usually taking longer if a child is older. You may be asked to provide photographs or a video, or to write a letter to the child before the first actual meeting. Should the match not feel right at this stage, it is important to raise the issue as soon as possible. You will also have the opportunity to meet those close to the child, and this may include members of the birth family.

Making adoption legal

Assuming all goes well, the child will be able to move in with you and during this time you will be visited at home by both your and the child's social workers over a period of weeks. No sooner than 10 weeks after the child has moved in with you (13 weeks in Scotland), you can apply to court for the adoption to become legal and the child's adoption certificate is issued. There may be a legal fee at this point, which is usually less than £150 and may be partially paid for by the local authority.

By law, the relevant local authority must provide support for adoptive families. This can be in a number of ways, including means-tested financial assistance, psychological support, and training and assistance if the placement disrupts (i.e. does not work out). Additionally, much support can be gained from the adoption agency as well as organizations such as Adoption UK and the British Association for Adoption & Fostering (see 'Useful addresses').

Statutory adoption leave

You may be entitled to statutory adoption leave of up to 52 weeks (of which 26 will be paid) if you have had 1 year's continuous service with your employer. In addition, you may be able to take 13 weeks unpaid leave (18 weeks if a child is disabled) up to 5 years after the child was placed. Your partner may also be able to take up to 2 weeks paternity leave (regardless of gender) within the first 56 days.

Adopting a child from abroad

Inter-country adoptions are becoming increasingly popular and there are many good reasons why this is so. Over 2200 children have been adopted from abroad since the year 2000, with nearly half coming from China. However, the implications of removing a child from his/her ethnic and cultural background have to be considered; as with domestic adoption, the interests of the child are paramount. The exact details of the procedures involved depends on the country from where the child is being adopted, although the assessment process for potential UK-based adopter(s) is the same as for UK adoptions. However, it is not unusual for the relevant authorities in the child's home country to require the potential adopter(s) to undergo that country's standard adoption assessment as well.

As described above, the first step is to register with a UK adoption agency and go through the assessment process. Once this has been completed, the Department for Children, Schools, and Families issues a Certificate of Eligibility to the relevant foreign authority. Matching with a child is performed within the relevant country. The details will vary from country to country and may be subject to particular conditions; for example, some countries require that the child has been available for adoption for a certain length of time before overseas adoption can be considered.

Once a potential match has been identified and discussed with the UK adoption agency, the prospective adopters can travel to meet the child. If the adoption is to proceed, the UK agency must be informed and they in turn notify the Department for Children, Schools, and Families who liaise with the relevant authorities in the child's country to confirm that the adoption can go ahead.

The child will need entry clearance in order to be brought into the UK. An adoption order from the country in question is required for this purpose, and, depending on the country, an additional UK adoption order may also be necessary. The local authority must be informed of the intention to apply for an adoption order within 14 days of the child entering the UK, and, consistent with the steps outlined above, social worker(s) will visit the home several times over the following weeks until the adoption order is made.

It is usual for charges to be payable for intercountry adoptions; for example, the UK adoption agency will probably charge for their involvement in the assessment process. Charges are also likely to be payable in the child's home country.

The Department for Children, Schools, and Families offers advice on intercountry adoption on its website (www.dfes.gov.uk/intercountry/adoption). Advice and links for specific countries are also available from this website. It is important to remember that the desirable adopter profile may well vary depending on the country in question and certain restrictions may be placed on particular groups who wish to adopt.

Case study

We decided to apply to be adoptive parents after three failed IVF attempts and 5 years of trying to have a child. Our infertility was unexplained and we could have had further treatments, but suddenly having our own genetic children didn't seem so important any more. We just wanted to be parents. We both worked with children and knew what wonderful beings they were. We were getting older and couldn't spend our thirties trying for children and then finding in our forties that it was too late to adopt.

The adoption preparation group nearly stopped us in our tracks as there was so much emphasis placed on how damaged the children were who were waiting to be adopted. The list of behaviours they could apparently exhibit were terrifying. It seemed that an adopted child would destroy our lives, not make them complete. Fortunately, we're both positive people and believed we had the will power required to love and nurture a child who had had a difficult start in life.

We had to wait 7 months before our overstretched social services department could find us an assessor. After a lengthy and intrusive assessment we were finally approved as adopters 14 months after attending our adoption preparation group. The process of assessment was one of the hardest things we have ever had to do—harder than IVF in fact, but in our case more successful.

Four months after being approved our social worker, who was very active in finding us a child, told us about a little boy who was just about to have his first birthday. He had only spent 6 months with his birth mother and had been thriving in a loving foster family for the previous 6 months. We were initially terrified as this was the closest we had come to being parents and we suddenly started to wonder whether we were really capable of it.

We carefully scrutinized all the information there was on our son to be. Both birth parents were known, as were most of the significant details in his short life. There was detailed medical information regarding his health and development and a few issues that worried us, but nothing that we thought we couldn't handle. We were officially matched with our son 2 weeks later and 6 weeks after that we met him for the first time. He was just 14 months old. My husband fell in love with him instantly. I just felt this strong need to care for this vulnerable little boy; love came later on for me.

After 10 days of introductions during which we gradually took on more care of our son we took him home with us for good. We were very anxious about uprooting him from the loving and supportive people who had become his family, and for a few days he appeared very unsure of himself and easily upset. This wasn't helped by a nasty stomach bug which he soon developed and kindly shared with our families who came to visit him. After the statutory wait, during which time we were visited and assessed weekly by social workers, we were allowed to adopt our son and no longer had to have contact with social services. By this time we couldn't remember life without him and I don't think he could remember life without us.

Life with our son has been an absolute dream come true. It is everything we hoped it would be and more. We cannot imagine loving a child more than we love him, and although he sometimes challenges us, as all children do, we never stop thinking how incredibly lucky we are to have him in our lives. He is such a pleasure to have around, he makes us laugh, smile, and wonder at the speed at which he learns and grows. A couple of weeks after he came to live with us we realized we had reached the point where we were actually glad we had been infertile and unable to have genetic children as they would never have measured up to the son we now have.

Useful addresses and further reading

Overview of fertility & the biological clock

Infertility Network UK
Charter House
43 St Leonards Road
Bexhill on Sea
East Sussex TN40 1JA
Tel 08701 188088
Fax 01424 731858
Email via the website www.infertilitynetworkuk.com

NICE guidelines on fertility
National Institute for Health and Clinical Excellence
MidCity Place
71 High Holborn
London WC1V 6NA
Tel 020 7067 5800
Fax 020 7067 5801
Email nice@nice.org.uk
Website www.nice.org.uk/

Getting pregnant.co.uk
Thinking about trying for a baby? Or already started trying?
www.gettingpregnant.co.co.uk/

Progress Educational Trust
This UK charity provides information and debate on assisted reproduction
and human genetics, promoting wider discussion.
Supported by the Department of Health.
Tel 020 7278 7870
www.progress.org.uk/

How to choose your clinic

Human Fertilisation and Embryology Authority
21 Bloomsbury Street
London WC1B 3HF
Tel 020 7291 8200
Fax 020 7291 8201
Email admin@hfea.gov.uk
Website www.hfea.gov.uk

The emotional side of infertility
British Infertility Counselling Association (BICA)
Offers information to patients seeking details of counsellors specializing in infertility
10 Alwyne Place
London N1 2NL
Tel 01372 451626
Email info@bica.net
Website www.bica.net

RELATE
Offers counselling for those seeking help with relationship difficulties
Premier House
Carolina Court
Lakeside
Doncaster
South Yorkshire DN4 1RA
Tel 0845 456 1310
Email relate@relate.org.uk

The NHS self help guides to Stress and Anxiety, Panic, Depression and Low Mood: available from your GP.

The Overcoming self-help guides use Cognitive Behavioural Therapy (CBT) techniques to treat disorders by changing unhelpful patterns of behaviour and thought. Many of the books are recommended by the Department of Health under the Books on Prescription scheme.

Overcoming panic
Overcoming depression
Overcoming low self esteem
Overcoming anger and irritability
Overcoming anxiety
Overcoming social anxiety and shyness
Published by Robinson Publishing
3 The Lanchester,
162 Fulham Palace Road,
London W6 9ER
Tel 020 8741 3663 Fax 020 8748 7562

Problems with Ovulation

Daisy Network
Premature menopause support group
The Daisy Network
PO Box 183
Rossendale
BB4 6WZ
Email daisy@daisynetwork.org.uk
Website www.daisynetwork.org.uk

Verity
The Polycystic Ovary Syndrome Self Help Group
Unit AS20.01
The Aberdeen Centre
22-24 Highbury Grove
London N5 2EA
Website verity-pcos.org.uk

Pre-implantation genetic tests

Genetic Interest Group
A national alliance of patient organisations which support children, families
and individuals affected by genetic disorders
Tel 020 7704 3141
Website www.gig.org.uk

Sperm or egg donation (Donor insemination)

Donor Conception Network (DC Network)

A self-help support group for those who are considering conception or have conceived with donor sperm or donor eggs

P.O. Box 7471

Nottingham NG3 6ZR

Tel 020 8245 4369

Fax 020 8245

Email enquiries@dcnetwork.org

Website www.dcnetwork.org/

National Gamete Donation Trust

A registered charity to raise awareness of and seek ways to alleviate the shortage of sperm, egg and embryo donors in the UK.

Tel 0845 226 9193

Website www.ngdt.co.uk/

Pink parents UK

Pink parents services to lesbian, gay, bisexual and transgendered families includes information and support to those who would like to have children.

Tel 08701 273 274

Website www.pinkparents.org.uk/

Single mother

A website for single mothers and those looking at their options or actively seeking to become one.

Website singlemother.typepad.com/

The gift of a child

This book describes the experiences of couples, individuals, parents and children who have had treatment or been conceived by donor insemination.

Written by Robert and Elizabeth Snowden of Exeter University.

Published by George Allen & Unwin 1993.

Available from

University of Exeter Press,

Reed Hall,

Streatham Drive, Exeter EX4 4QR.

Tel 01392 263066

Email uep@ex.ac.uk

Telling and Talking

'Telling' and Talking about Donor Conception with 0-7 year olds. A guide for parents by Olivia Montuschi published by Donor Conception Network.

Donor Conception Network (DC Network)

P.O. Box 7471

Nottingham NG3 6ZR

Tel 020 8245 4369

Email enquiries@dcnetwork.org

Surrogacy

Childlessness overcome through surrogacy (COTS)

Chairperson Kim Cotton,

4 The Fairway,

New Barnet,

Herts EN5 1HN

Email cotsuk@enterprise.net

Website www.surrogacy.org.uk/

For further information on parental orders for surrogacy:

Department of Health

Health Promotion Division

Room 417

Wellington House

133-155 Waterloo Road

London SE1 8UG

Tel 020 7972 2000

Surrogacy UK

A website and message board providing advice on surrogacy in the UK.

Tel 01531 821889

Website www.surrogacyuk.org/

Gynaecological problems and fertility

Endometriosis UK

50 Westminster Palace Gardens

Artillery Row

London SW1P 1RL

Tel 020 7222 2776

Website www.endometriosis-uk.org/

Pregnancy after fertility treatment

AceBabes
Offers support on pregnancy following fertility treatment
P.O. Box 6979
Derby DE1 9HY
Tel 0845 838 1593
Email enquiries@acebabes.co.uk
Website www.acebabes.co.uk/

Multiple Births Foundation
Provides professional support and information about all aspects of multiple births.
The Multiple Births Foundation
Hammersmith House level 4
Queen Charlotte's & Chlesea Hospital
Du Cane Road
London W12 0HS
Tel 020 8383 3519
Fax 020 8383 3041
Email info@multiplebirths.org.uk
Website multiplebirths.org.uk

Ectopic Pregnancy Trust
Maternity Unit
The Hillingdon Hospital
Pield Heath Road
Uxbridge
Middlesex UB8 3NN
Tel 01895 238025
Email ept@ectopic.org.uk
Website ectopic.org.uk/

Miscarriage Association
Care of Clayton Hospital
Northgate Wakefield
West Yorkshire WF1 3JS
Tel 01924 200799 (Monday–Friday 9-4)
Website miscarriageassociation.org.uk/

Association of Early Pregnancy Units
for details of your nearest Early Pregnancy Unit
Website www.earlypregnancy.org.uk

Royal College of Obstetricians & Gynaecologists
Patient information on all aspects of pregnancy
Royal College of Obstetricians & Gynaecologists
27 Sussex Place
Regent's Park
London NW1 4RG
Tel 020 7772 6200
www.rcog.org.uk

Coping with infertility

More to Life
A national support network providing a service for people exploring what life without children has to offer.
Tel 08701 188 088

Beyond childlessness. For every woman who wanted to have a child – and didn't
Authors Rachel Black and Louise Scull 2005
Rodale International Ltd,
7-10 Chandos Street,
London W1G 9AD
Website www.rodale.co.uk

Adoption

Adoption Register for England and Wales
Unit 4 Pavilion Business Park
Royds Hall Road
Wortley
Leeds LS12 6AJ
Tel 0870 750 2173
Website www.adoptionregister.org.uk

Adoption UK
46 The Green
South Bar Street
Banbury OX16 9AB
Tel 01295 752240
Fax 01295 752241
Website www.adoptionuk.com/

Consortium of Voluntary Adoption Agencies
14 Liverpool Street
Chester CH2 1AE
Tel 01767 652153
Website www.cvaa.org.uk

British Association for Adoption & Fostering
Head Office
Saffron House
6-10 Kirby Street
London EC1N 8TS
There are also Country and Regional Offices – addresses available on the
website or from Head Office
Tel 020 7421 2600
Website www.baaf.org.uk

Intercountry Adoption Centre
64-66 High Street
Barnet
Hertfordshire EN5 5SJ
Tel 0870 516 8742
Website www.icacentre.org.uk

Parent information service
An organisation providing help and support, for those with any queries
concerning adoption
P.P.I.S.
Lower Boddington
Daventry
Northants NN11 6YB
Tel 01327 260195 11am - 4pm weekdays

Glossary

Adhesions Internal scar tissue usually formed as a result of surgery or infection.

Adrenal gland Small hormone-producing organ located above each kidney. Produces the hormones cortisol and aldosterone.

Amniocentesis Fluid from around the fetus (the amniotic fluid) can be sampled using a needle and syringe. Fetal cells contained in this fluid can be tested to check if the fetus carries the correct number of chromosomes. The most common reason for an amniocentesis is to check if the fetus has an extra chromosome 21, known as Down syndrome. If one of the parents is known to carry a genetic disorder, it is possible to test the fetus in this way if the genetic defect (mutation) has been identified. It is usually done at 16 weeks of pregnancy, but can be done later. It carries a small risk of miscarriage (approximately 0.5 per cent).

Amenorrhoea Absence of menstruation.

AMH (anti-Müllerian hormone) Hormone produced by ovarian follicles which can be measured in the blood and indirectly reflects the number of follicles in the ovary. Often used to help predict the response to IVF.

Aneuploidy Abnormal number of chromosomes (usually one too many or one too few).

Anovulation Failure to release an egg from the ovary.

Antral follicle count Number of follicles that are visible on an ultrasound scan of the ovary.

Blastocyst A stage in the development of the embryo about 5 days after fertilization. The cluster of dividing cells becomes hollow, with the outer cells destined to form the placenta or afterbirth, with an 'inner cell mass' which will form the fetus and eventually all the tissues of the body.

BMI (body mass index) Measure of weight in relation to height. Calculated as weight in kilograms/(height in metres)^2.

Caesarean section Operation to deliver a baby, usually done via a bikini line scar. May be planned ('elective') or unexpected ('emergency'). Often abbreviated to LSCS (lower segment Caesarean section).

Cell Basic unit of all living organisms.

Cervix Neck of the uterus (womb).

Chromosome Structure made of DNA containing genetic information. All human cells, apart from mature eggs and sperm, contain 23 pairs of chromosomes including either two X chromosomes (female) or one X and one Y chromosome (male). Mature eggs and sperm contain half that number (23 chromosomes including one X or one Y chromosome).

Clomifene (clomifene citrate or Clomid) Fertility drug that makes the pituitary gland release more follicle-stimulating hormone (FSH) which then stimulates the growth of follicles in the ovary.

CMV (cytomegalovirus) Common virus related to herpes. Most infections do not cause any symptoms, although there may be a flu-like illness. Can be harmful to unborn babies if the mother catches CMV when pregnant. Most adults have caught CMV in childhood and so are immune to further infection. There is no vaccine available.

Corpus luteum Once the egg has been released from the follicle, the follicle changes into a structure called the corpus luteum which produces the hormone progesterone.

CVS (chorionic villus sampling) A sample of the placenta is taken using a needle which is usually passed through the mother's tummy. Sometimes, depending on the position of the placenta, the needle is passed through the cervix. It is usually done after 12 weeks of pregnancy and can be used to examine the number of chromosomes the fetus has. If one of the parents is known to carry a genetic disorder, it is possible to test the fetus in this way if the genetic defect (mutation) has been identified. It carries a slightly higher risk of miscarriage than amniocentesis, but can be done a month earlier in the pregnancy.

D&C Dilatation and curettage: dilatation of the cervix and curettage of uterine cavity. Sometimes called a 'scrape'.

Deep vein thrombosis (DVT) Clot that forms in the vein of a leg, usually causing painful swelling of the calf and/or thigh. May lead to a pulmonary embolus, where a piece of a blood clot lodges in the lungs (a serious medical problem).

Diabetes A disorder when the body is unable to control the levels of sugar in the blood. Type 1 diabetes usually starts in children or young adults and is the result of the pancreas being unable to produce enough insulin. Type 2 diabetes usually starts later in life and is the result of the body's cells becoming resistant to the effects of insulin. It is more common if overweight (particularly in women with polycystic ovary syndrome) and when there is a family history of diabetes. Diabetes can also occur only in pregnancy; this is called gestational diabetes (GDM).

Dominant follicle At the beginning of each menstrual cycle, a small number of follicles begin to grow. The largest follicle begins to suppress the growth of its competitors and is called the dominant follicle. This is the follicle from which the egg will be released (ovulation).

Down syndrome Lifelong condition due to the presence of an extra chromosome 21 which causes learning difficulties.

Embryo Once fertilized, the egg is known as an embryo until the 10th week of pregnancy when it is called the fetus.

Endometriosis Condition where cells that are the same as those lining the uterus are found elsewhere in the pelvis (and rarely beyond the pelvis). These cells bleed on a monthly basis, which can cause pain and the formation of scar tissue. Infertility can result from the scar tissue formed by endometriosis, although it is not clear if minor degrees of endometriosis affect fertility.

Endometrium Lining of the uterus (womb).

Epididymis The epididymis is a very coiled tube which sits on top of the testis. Sperm are stored and matured in the epididymis.

ERPC (evacuation of retained products of conception) Operation to empty the uterus (womb) after a miscarriage.

Fetus Unborn baby.

Fallopian tubes Pair of tubes, one leading from each ovary into the uterus, which transport the egg and sperm. Site of fertilization.

Follicle Structure in the ovary that contains the egg. Growing follicles have a fluid centre and can be seen on an ultrasound scan as a black circle.

FSH (follicle-stimulating hormone) Hormone released from the pituitary that stimulates the growth of follicles in the ovary.

Gene Unit of inheritance. There are always two copies of a gene, one inherited from the mother and one from the father. Genes are coded for by DNA which forms the chromosomes.

GIFT (gamete intra-Fallopian transfer) Fertility treatment where eggs are collected in the same way as for IVF and are transferred into one of the Fallopian tubes together with some sperm in an operation called a laparoscopy.

Gonadotrophins Collective term for the hormones that can stimulate the ovaries or testes (follicle-stimulating hormone, luteinizing hormone, human chorionic gonadotrophin).

GnRH (gonadotrophin-releasing hormone) Hormone produced by a part of the brain called the hypothalamus which stimulates the release of follicle-stimulating hormone and luteinizing hormone.

hCG (human chorionic gonadotrophin, also known as beta-hCG) Hormone usually produced by the placenta. It can be measured in the blood or urine to detect pregnancy. May be given as an injection to trigger ovulation.

Hepatitis B Virus that is carried in the blood and body fluids which may result in liver damage, although most of those infected will have no symptoms. The virus can be caught by contact with infected blood or body fluids and can be passed from mother to baby during childbirth. There is a vaccine to protect against the virus.

Hepatitis C Virus that is carried in the blood and body fluids which may result in liver damage. Infection is usually spread by contact with infected blood rather than with other body fluids. It can also be passed from mother to baby during childbirth. There is no vaccine against hepatitis C at present.

HFEA (Human Fertilisation and Embryology Authority) Regulator of most forms of fertility treatment in the UK.

HIV (human immunodeficiency virus) HIV is an infection carried in the blood and body fluids of an infected person. It can be spread by contact with these fluids and can also be passed from mother to baby during childbirth. The virus causes weakening of the immune system and acquired immune deficiency syndrome (AIDS), now usually called HIV disease. No vaccine is available at present.

Hormone Chemical messenger released into the bloodstream by an organ called a gland.

Hyperstimulation of the ovary Hormonal stimulation of the ovary to produce more than one mature follicle at a time. Controlled hyperstimulation is used for superovulation and IVF.

Hypothalamus Central part of the brain that integrates internal and external influences and may indirectly affect ovarian and testicular function.

Hysteroscopy Investigation to examine the cavity of the uterus (womb). It involves passing a fine camera through the vagina and cervix into the uterus. The procedure can be done awake as an outpatient or more commonly under a general anaesthetic as a day case.

ICSI (intra-cytoplasmic sperm injection) Form of IVF where a single sperm is injected into a single egg to assist fertilization.

IVIG (immunoglobulin) Concentrated antibody preparation used to provide short-term protection against specific conditions. Antibodies are proteins produced by the immune system to neutralize foreign molecules such as viruses and bacteria.

Inhibin B Hormone produced by ovarian follicles that can be measured in a blood test to provide an estimate of the number of follicles in the ovary.

IUI (intra-uterine insemination) Fertility treatment where concentrated sperm is introduced into the uterus using a fine straw which is passed through the cervix at the time of ovulation.

IVF (*in vitro* fertilization) Fertility treatment where the egg and the sperm are mixed together outside the body. Embryos resulting from this treatment can be transferred into the uterus (womb).

Laparoscopy Operation to examine the inside of the abdomen and pelvis with a special camera inserted just below the belly button (umbilicus).

LMP (last menstrual period) Date that the last period *started* (not finished).

LH (luteinizing hormone) Hormone produced by the pituitary gland that triggers ovulation.

Menopause Last ever menstrual period.

Microsurgery Form of surgery where the surgeon looks through a special operating microscope to magnify the structures being operated on.

Miscarriage Loss of a pregnancy before 24 weeks.

Mittelschmerz Pelvic pain associated with ovulation.

NHS (National Health Service) State-funded health service in the UK.

Oestradiol Naturally occurring form of oestrogen.

Oestrogen Hormone produced by growing follicles in the ovary.

Omphalocele Defect in the abdominal wall of a fetus or baby where the umbilical cord inserts. The defect, which is covered by a membrane, usually contains loops of bowel.

OHSS (ovarian hyperstimulation syndrome) Uncontrolled over-stimulation of the ovaries associated with pooling of fluid within the abdominal cavity and sometimes around the lungs. Also associated with an increased risk of developing a clot in the legs (deep vein thrombosis (DVT)) or on the lungs (pulmonary embolus (PE)).

Ovarian reserve Concept which broadly refers to the number of eggs remaining in the ovary and their quality, or potential to become a baby.

Ovulation Release of an egg from a mature dominant follicle.

Ovulation induction Treatment to make the ovary release an egg.

PID (pelvic inflammatory disease) Infection of the Fallopian tubes and uterus, as opposed to a vaginal infection such as thrush (candida) or bacterial vaginosis (BV).

Penis Male external sex organ.

Pituitary gland Hormone-producing part of the brain located between the eyes. Produces the hormones that control the production of eggs and sperm amongst others.

Placenta Structure formed as part of the pregnancy that supplies the fetus with oxygen and nutrients taken from the mother's blood. Sometimes called the afterbirth as it is delivered after the baby.

PCO (polycystic ovaries) Ovaries which contain an increased number of follicles and are usually larger than the average size. The majority of women with PCO will not have polycystic ovary syndrome (PCOS).

PCOS (polycystic ovary syndrome) A condition where affected women have polycystic ovaries together with irregular periods, acne, or an increased amount of male pattern hair growth on their face or body.

Pouch of Douglas Area of the pelvis that lies internally behind the cervix and vagina but in front of the rectum (back passage).

Pre-eclampsia Common complication of the last 3 months of pregnancy when the mother's blood pressure rises and she develops protein in her urine. The mother may become severely ill and may even have a fit (known as eclampsia). In addition, the fetus may be affected and may not grow as well as it should. The only treatment for this condition is to deliver the baby. If the mother's blood pressure is very high, she may be given treatment to control it until it is possible to deliver the baby.

PGD (preimplantation genetic diagnosis) Removal of one or two cells from an embryo that has been created by IVF to test for a known genetic disorder. If there is an embryo free from the condition in question, it can be selected for transfer into the uterus (womb).

PGS (preimplantation genetic screening) Removal of one or two cells from an embryo that has been created by IVF to check the number of chromosomes.

Premature labour Labour before 37 weeks of pregnancy.

PCT (primary care trust) Regional NHS funding body.

Primary infertility The person in question has never been pregnant.

Progesterone Hormone produced by the collapsed follicle (now called the corpus luteum) which is left after the egg has been released (ovulation). Progesterone prepares the endometrium for pregnancy should it occur. The hormone level decreases if pregnancy has not occurred and a period results.

Prolactin Hormone produced by the pituitary gland which promotes milk production during breast feeding. High levels can stop ovulation.

Rubella Virus spread by coughs and sneezes otherwise known as german measles. May be harmful to the unborn baby if the mother is infected during pregnancy. All women planning pregnancy should ensure that they are immune, which can be checked with a blood test.

Secondary infertility Person who has had at least one pregnancy but has had a delay in conceiving again.

Selective reduction See selective termination.

Selective termination Procedure where one or more of the fetuses within a multiple pregnancy are stopped from developing further by giving a lethal injection. May be dangerous for the remaining fetus(es). Also known as selective reduction.

Speculum Instrument made of plastic or metal which is inserted into the vagina in order to visualize the cervix.

Spina bifida Developmental abnormality of the spine (a neural tube defect) where the bony part has gaps in it, exposing the spinal cord. The condition varies from very minor, with affected individuals being unaware of it, to severe when the spinal cord may become damaged.

Steroids Naturally occurring steroids are hormones made from cholesterol, such as cortisol, oestrogens, progesterone, and testosterone. Artificial steroids can also be given to treat various medical conditions, particularly when it is necessary to damp down the immune system.

Superovulation Fertility treatment to make the ovary produce more than one egg at ovulation.

Surrogacy One woman (the surrogate) carries a pregnancy for another, giving her the baby at birth.

Testes/testicles Male organ where sperm is made. There are two testicles ('balls') which are found in a sac (scrotum) either side of the base of the penis.

Testosterone Male hormone predominantly produced by the testicles in men. Women also produce a small amount from the ovaries.

Thrombosis Blood clot. Two serious forms are deep vein thrombosis (DVT) where the clot forms in the vein of a leg, and pulmonary embolus (PE), where a piece of a blood clot lodges in the lungs.

Ultrasound High-frequency sound waves used to make images of internal organs. The probe used to make these images may be put over the area of interest (e.g. on the abdomen), but more commonly for fertility investigations a special thin probe is put into the vagina in order to visualize the uterus and ovaries in detail.

Uterus (womb) The uterus usually tilts forward (known as an anteverted uterus) but in 15 per cent of women it tilts backwards (retroverted uterus). The tilt does not affect fertility.

Vas deferens Tubes that carry sperm from the testicles to the penis.

ZIFT (zygote intra-Fallopian transfer) Form of IVF where the zygote (a one-cell embryo) is transferred into the Fallopian tube.

Index